Orthodontics for Dental Hygienists and Dental Therapists

# Orthodontics for Dental Hygienists and Dental Therapists

*Tina Raked*

**WILEY** Blackwell

*Registered Offices*
John Wiley & Sons, Inc., 111 River Street, Hoboken, NJ 07030, USA
John Wiley & Sons Ltd, The Atrium, Southern Gate, Chichester, West Sussex, PO19 8SQ, UK

*Editorial Office*
9600 Garsington Road, Oxford, OX4 2DQ, UK

For details of our global editorial offices, customer services, and more information about Wiley products visit us at www.wiley.com.

Wiley also publishes its books in a variety of electronic formats and by print-on-demand. Some content that appears in standard print versions of this book may not be available in other formats.

*Library of Congress Cataloging-in-Publication Data*

Names: Raked, Tina, author.
Title: Orthodontics for dental hygienists and dental therapists / Tina Raked.
Description: Hoboken, NJ : Wiley, 2017. | Includes bibliographical references and index. |
Identifiers: LCCN 2017024245 (print) | LCCN 2017024900 (ebook) | ISBN 9781119251897 (pdf) |
    ISBN 9781119251866 (epub) | ISBN 9781119251880 (pbk.)
Subjects: | MESH: Orthodontics | Dental Auxiliaries
Classification: LCC RK521 (ebook) | LCC RK521 (print) | NLM WU 400 | DDC 617.6/43–dc23
LC record available at https://lccn.loc.gov/2017024245

Cover design: Wiley
Cover image: Courtesy of Tina Raked

Set in 10/12pt Warnock by SPi Global, Pondicherry, India
Printed and bound in Malaysia by Vivar Printing Sdn Bhd

10 9 8 7 6 5 4 3 2 1

*To my parents and my family for their love, encouragement and endless support.*

# Contents

## Preface

As an oral health therapist, I am grateful to have this opportunity to help oral health and dental hygiene students to gain a better understanding of the fundamentals of orthodontic theories and gain elementary clinical guidance. My aim is to provide a textbook that breaks down the orthodontic mechanics and delivers explanations of the basic orthodontic theories in a simple approach. This book is intended for all undergraduate dental hygiene, dental therapy and oral health students.

Among various countries the role and scope of practice of oral health therapists, dental hygienists and dental therapists greatly varies. Nevertheless, it is best to have validations on scopes of practice with the dental associations within each state or country to confirm the clinical limitations prior to any clinical practice.

To become valuable team members in an orthodontic practice, it is crucial to understand the orthodontic mechanics and fundamentals regardless of the clinical limitations. This allows therapists to communicate better with patients and other colleagues. Hence, it is important that all oral health therapists, dental hygienists and dental therapists have the essential theoretical knowledge of the field to be able to understand the clinical outcomes and treatments carried out by orthodontists.

Tina Raked
Sydney, Australia
2017

## Acknowledgements

It was an honour to have the guidance of Professor Ali Darendeliler (Chair of the Discipline of Orthodontics at the Faculty of Dentistry in Sydney and Head of Sydney Dental Hospital's Department of Orthodontics). I am very grateful to the following orthodontists for their support, who kindly contributed patient cases: Dr Jim Bokas, Dr Kit Chan, Dr Nour Eldin Tarraf, Dr Shimanto K. Purkayastha. I am very grateful to Gosia Olas for all her hard work and effort for the illustrations and a special thanks to Mehran Iranloo for contributing to the illustrations for Chapter 2 and Joanna Culley for Chapter 4 illustrations.

## About the Companion Website

Remember to visit the companion website for this book:

**www.wiley.com/go/raked/orthodontics_dental_hygienists**

There you will find valuable material designed to enhance your learning, including:

- Multiple choice questions with answers.

Scan this QR code to visit the companion website.

1

## Scope of Practice and Competency

Dental care services may require a team of dental professionals to carry out the necessary treatments. There are several divisions for registered dental practitioners in different types of healthcare settings with diverse scopes of practice based on their training, education and competence. These divisions in the dental industry vary greatly between countries.

### Dentists

Dentists are independent practitioners with a range of responsibilities associated with assessment, prevention, diagnosis, treatment and management of dental lesions, deformities, traumas and diseases of human teeth and associated structures. Care is provided to patients of all ages. Dentists can practise all aspects of dentistry that is within their education, training and competency and can further pursue a specialist training to become dental specialists in various fields of dentistry. Examples of these specialties include:

- orthodontics
- endodontics
- oral and maxillofacial surgery
- oral pathology
- oral surgery
- periodontics
- paediatric dentistry
- prosthodontics
- special needs dentistry.

### Oral Health Therapists

This dual-qualified programme provides graduates with sufficient knowledge of all aspects of dental hygiene and dental therapy. In a general dental setting, the scope is to provide assessment, diagnosis and treatment for children and adolescents, working closely with dentists. Depending on the national board approved programme, the

*Orthodontics for Dental Hygienists and Dental Therapists*, First Edition. Tina Raked.
© 2018 John Wiley & Sons Ltd. Published 2018 by John Wiley & Sons Ltd.
Companion website: www.wiley.com/go/raked/orthodontics_dental_hygienists

treatment can be carried out for patients of all ages. The scope is regulated to preventative services, restorative work and fillings, extraction of deciduous teeth, treatment of periodontal diseases, oral health education and promotion. Oral health therapists work closely with specialists in an orthodontic setting to carry out the treatment plan designed by the orthodontist. Based on the training and education provided in the programme, the level of competency greatly varies.

## Dental Hygienists

Assessment, diagnosis, treatment and management of mild to moderate periodontal diseases are the primary roles of dental hygienists. Treating severe periodontal cases with a surgical approach is beyond the scope of dental hygienists. In these instances, dental hygienists work closely with periodontists to manage the condition. The main role is oral health education and prevention of oral diseases in patients of all ages, by promoting better oral health and hygiene. In a general dental setting, dental hygienists only work within a structured professional relationship with dentists. In the orthodontic setting, dental hygienists work under the guidance and supervision of an orthodontist.

## Dental Therapists

The primary role of the dental therapist is assessment, diagnosis and management of dental caries. This is achieved by providing preventative care services, pulpotomies and extraction of deciduous teeth, restorative procedures for children and adolescents. Depending on the national board approved programmes, the age limits vary and some scopes allow treatment for patients of all ages. One of the key roles of dental therapists is enhancing better oral health with oral health promotion and education for patients of all ages. Dental therapists are only permitted to work within a structured professional relationship established with dentists.

## Orthodontic Treatment

The scope of orthodontics is not narrowed solely to straightening teeth. The field of orthodontics is about treatment of irregularities in growth and development of the orofacial complex, enhancing function and aesthetics. Orthodontic treatment contributes to improving the physical and mental wellbeing of the patient. A team approach by dental professionals is needed to achieve successful outcomes and to provide the patient with a pleasant experience. Some cases may require a team of specialists cooperating together to guide the patient towards their orthodontic goal and providing them with a balanced facial appearance, healthy periodontium and a functional occlusion with an aesthetically pleasing smile.

In an orthodontic practice, oral health therapists, dental therapists and dental hygienists work closely with orthodontists to carry out the treatment plan under the supervision of the specialist. The level of training of dental practitioners varies greatly worldwide. Thus, for efficient and quality dental treatment, it is critical to confirm the limitations and scope of practice within each state or country before any form of clinical practice. Oral health therapists, dental hygienists and dental therapists can be valuable team members in an orthodontic setting, but they also play an important role in general dental clinics. A greater knowledge of orthodontics is therefore essential for these practitioners to help to monitor dental growth and development closely during regular dental visits and to make appropriate referrals as required.

Every orthodontist will manage their patients differently based on their education and training. Over the years, there have been well-known specialists who have contributed to the evolution of orthodontics by introducing advanced and contemporary techniques and appliances. There can be numerous ways to reach a common goal using various treatment options and appliances. These goals may not always be what the specialist considers as the norm or ideal. The treatment objective is to address the chief complaint and to respect the goals and objectives requested by the patient.

There is sufficient knowledge and understanding of the ideal occlusion. One scheme that is well known and used as guidance by many specialists is Andrews' six keys (Andrews, 1972). An ideal occlusion is shown in Figure 1.1. The six keys are as follows:

1) Correct molar relationship
2) Correct crown angulation
3) Correct crown inclination
4) No rotations
5) No spaces
6) Flat occlusal plane.

A variety of treatment options can be outlined to reach the desired goals. These goals and procedures must be discussed in depth and approved by the patient. A treatment plan may indicate the need or combination of the following:

- extractions
- functional appliances (influences dentoalveolar and muscular changes)

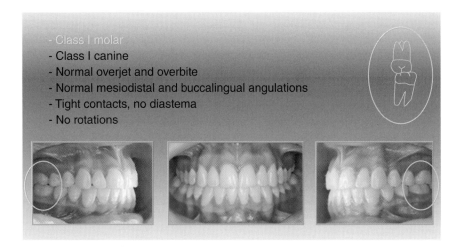

Figure 1.1 Normal occlusion. *Source*: Courtesy of Professor Ali Darendeliler.

- orthopaedic appliances (stimulate bone growth and position)
- removable appliances
- full/partial upper and lower fixed appliances
- single arch fixed appliances
- orthognathic surgery
- acceptance of the malocclusion.

Typically, treatment in deciduous dentition is not indicated and is delayed until early mixed dentition, with an exception for significant facial asymmetry and craniofacial deformities. Early treatment aids in minimising the severity of the orthodontic problem and reduces the need for complex treatment once the permanent dentition is established. Adults of all ages can undergo treatment, depending on the health of the underlying periodontium. In severe cases, orthodontic therapy alone may not suffice and a combination of orthognathic surgery and restorative dental procedures may be needed, particularly if growth has ceased. In some instances, patients may choose to accept their orthodontic problem and may not seek treatment. Acceptance of the malocclusion or skeletal disharmony is always an option if the patient disagrees with all the treatment options provided by the specialist. Growth and development, orthodontic assessment, treatment planning and various appliances are discussed in the remaining chapters in this book.

## Orthodontic Indices

Several orthodontic indices have been developed to create a better understanding of the severity of the orthodontic problem and the need for treatment. Some of the commonly used indices include the Index of Orthodontics Treatment Need (1987), the Peer Assessment Rating and the Index of Complexity Outcome and Need.

The Index of Orthodontic Treatment Need (Daniels and Richmond, 2000) is designed for children under the age of 18 years. There are two components to this index. The first is the dental health element and the second is aesthetics. The British Orthodontic Society provides five grades that allow clinicians to evaluate the rationale for treatment. The aesthetic aspect of this index employs a series of ten photographs. The index only assesses the incisors and does not consider all possible malocclusions, such as class III and open bites.

The Peer Assessment Rating (Richmond et al., 1992) was developed to assess the effectiveness and success of the orthodontic treatment outcome based on various occlusal traits. The traits assessed include crowding, buccal segment relationships, overjet, overbite and midlines. Each trait is given a score and the diagnosis of severity is made based on the total of the scores.

The Index of complexity Outcome and Need is the combination of scores from the Index of Orthodontic Treatment Need and the Peer Assessment Rating. The final scores indicate the severity of the orthodontic issue and the need for treatment. Score of more than 43 indicates a need for treatment. Other commonly used indices include the Treatment Priority Index (Grainger, 1967) and Dental Aesthetic Index (Cons et al., 1987).

## References

Andrews, L. F., The six keys to normal occlusion. *Am J Orthod*, 1972; 62(3): 296–309.

Cons, N. C., Jenny, J., Kohout, K. DAI: The dental aesthetic index. *Am J Orthod Dentofacial Orthop*, 1987; 92(6): 521–522.

Daniels, C., Richmond, S. The development of the Index of Complexity, Outcome and Need (ICON). *Br J Orthod*, 2000; 27: 149–162.

Grainger, R. M. Orthodontic treatment priority index. *Vital Health Stat* 2, 1967; (25): 1–49.

Richmond, S., Shaw, W. C., O'Brien, K. D., et al. The development of the PAR Index (Peer Assessment Rating): reliability and validity. *Eur J Orthod*, 1992; 14(2): 125–139.

## Further Reading

Dental Board of Australia. Guidelines for scope of practice. 30 June 2014. Available at http://www.dentalboard.gov.au/Codes-Guidelines/Policies-Codes-Guidelines/Guidelines-Scope-of-practice.aspx (accessed 4 April 2017).

Jones, M. L., Oliver, R. G. *W & H Orthodontic Notes*. 6th ed. Oxford: Wright; 2000.

Mitchell, L. *An Introduction to Orthodontics*. 3rd ed. Oxford: Oxford University Press; 2007.

# 2

# Growth and Development

## Craniofacial Growth and Development

A better understanding of growth and development can create an easy path in gaining superior knowledge of diseases and abnormal developmental processes. In some cases, early detection of abnormalities can prevent complex treatments. This chapter provides a brief summary of craniofacial growth and tooth development.

### What is Growth?

Over the years, there have been several definitions and justifications of growth. Some refer to growth as an increase in the size or number or changes in the amount of living substance occurring in a process of development.

Human growth refers to numerous sequential, developmental stages involving tissue and cell differentiations for formation of various organs and systems. Development is an evolutionary process from initiation to maturation. However, growth and development are not always about an increase in size or multiplication of cells. In some cases, certain cells and tissues must differentiate, change or decrease in size or number for other cells to form completely without abnormalities; for example, if remnant cells (remaining cells) persist during development and differentiation, they may result in cysts and complicate the growth process.

### What Factors Affect Growth?

Several factors can influence growth. These factors can be categorised into two major groups of genetics and environmental. Hereditary factors or genetics play a significant role in regulating growth patterns. Thus, people are distinct because of their unique genetic make-up and individualised growth and development. Environmental dynamics can modify the outcomes of normal growth patterns depending on the time and type of environmental influence. Human growth consists of two phases of prenatal (before birth) and postnatal (after birth).

## Prenatal Developmental Phases

The normal human prenatal development consists of three phases, beginning with fertilisation and proceeding to formation of the three germ layers (ectoderm, mesoderm and endoderm). The first three weeks are considered to be the first prenatal phase. From the fourth prenatal week, the second phase initiates and extends to the eighth week. Any disturbances during the second prenatal phase may lead to various abnormalities and defects, depending on the type and timing of the disruption. This period is vital, as the three germ cells differentiate into several tissues and gives rise to the organs and systems. The prenatal development ends with the fetal phase, from the ninth to the fortieth week. The focus of this chapter is on the first two stages of prenatal development and provides a summary of postnatal craniofacial growth.

### First Prenatal Phase (Weeks 1–3)

Embryogenesis is the term given to the process of embryo formation and development (Figure 2.1). An embryo development begins with a zygote formation in a process called fertilisation. Sperm swim through the fallopian tube until they reach the ovum (egg) that has been released from one of the ovaries. Sperm attack the ovum to break through the physical barriers and membranes for its nuclei to fuse with the egg nuclei to form a zygote (Figure 2.2). The zygote travels towards the uterus, down the fallopian tube.

The zygote undergoes several mitotic cell divisions during a process called cleavage and develops into a ball of cells known as the morula. Three days after fertilisation, the morula enters the uterus. The outer cells of the morula undergo compaction within a week and the morula becomes a blastocyst. It consists of a single outer layer called the trophoblast and a fluid-filled space, the blastocoel (also known as the blastocyst cavity). There are groups of cells inside the trophoblast, called the inner cell mass or embryoblast.

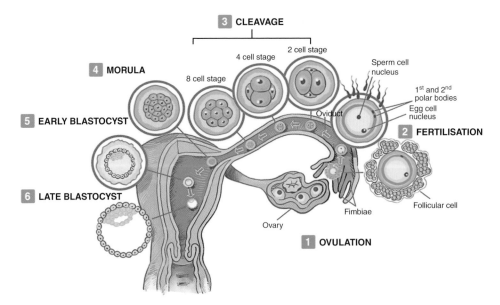

Figure 2.1 The first prenatal phase (weeks 1–3).

Implantation of the blastocyst occurs as it adheres to the endometrium (the mucous membrane lining of the uterus) by the end of the first week. The inner cell mass gives rise to the embryo by forming a bilaminar disc. The bilaminar disc is composed of two layers:

1) Epiblasts: give rise to the three germ cells.
2) Hypoblasts: form the outer embryonic membrane responsible for protection of the embryo and the supply of nutrition.

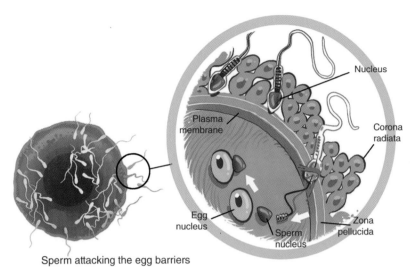

Figure 2.2 Fertilisation.

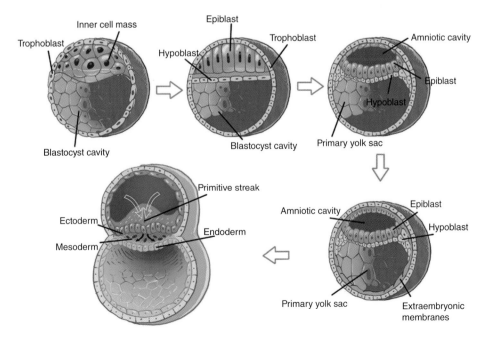

Figure 2.3 Gastrulation.

During the second week, an amniotic cavity develops and the blastocyst cavity becomes the primary yolk sac. The amniotic cavity is located within the inner cell mass and contains amniotic fluid, which is crucial for the embryo.

Gastrulation is a critical phase that occurs three weeks after fertilisation (Figure 2.3). This process gives rise to the three germ cells (Box 2.1). This stage of embryo development begins with the formation of the primitive streak. The primitive streak is a groove on the midline of the epiblast that occurs due to thickening of the peripheral surfaces. This determines the embryo axis. The bilaminar disc then develops into a trilaminar disc by a series of cell invaginations (cell infolding). The primitive streak widens and

---

**Box 2.1  Derivatives of Germ Layers**

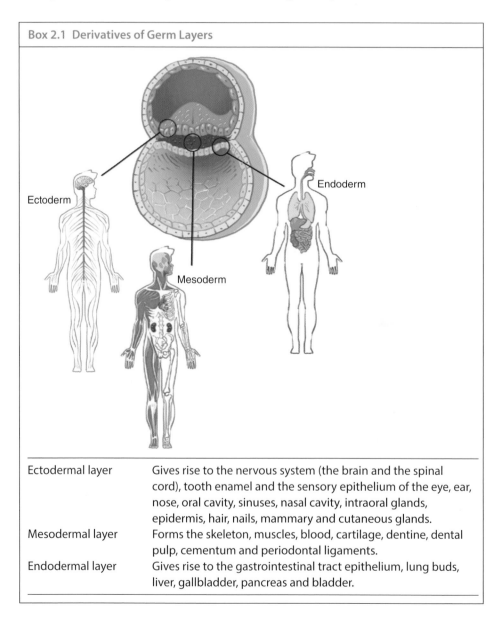

| | |
|---|---|
| Ectodermal layer | Gives rise to the nervous system (the brain and the spinal cord), tooth enamel and the sensory epithelium of the eye, ear, nose, oral cavity, sinuses, nasal cavity, intraoral glands, epidermis, hair, nails, mammary and cutaneous glands. |
| Mesodermal layer | Forms the skeleton, muscles, blood, cartilage, dentine, dental pulp, cementum and periodontal ligaments. |
| Endodermal layer | Gives rise to the gastrointestinal tract epithelium, lung buds, liver, gallbladder, pancreas and bladder. |

cells from the epiblast move towards the hypoblast and eventually replace the hypoblast cells to form the endoderm. The cells that move between the epiblast and the endoderm become the mesoderm. By this stage, the invagination of epiblast cells from the primitive streak ceases. The remaining epiblast cells become the ectoderm and are located above the mesodermal layer.

### Second Prenatal Phase (Week 4–8)

Upon formation of the germ layers, a neural plate and a neural tube forms via a folding process called neurulation (Figure 2.4). A flexible rod-shaped body known as the notochord, located beneath the ectodermal layer, induces ectoderm thickening. The notochord is a mesoderm derivative and induces neural plate formation. The growth of the neural plate begins from the cranial (head of the embryo) to the caudal (tail of the embryo). These regions determine the future brain position at the cranial and the spinal cord towards the caudal. The embryo is termed neurula at this stage of development.

The lateral borders of the neural plate elevate and fold to meet in the midline. This action results in the neural groove development. At the beginning of the fourth prenatal week, the neural fold fuses and forms the neural tube. Neurulation is finalised when the neural folds completely fuse and detach from the ectoderm. The central nervous system ascends from the neural tube. Neural crests are cells that develop surrounding the neural tube and will give rise to the peripheral nervous system.

Four weeks after fertilisation, somites develop in paired bodies from the mesodermal cell layer. Somites are found along the neural tube and eventually give rise to the skeleton and muscles. During these structural changes, the developing heart is pushed beneath the brain and the stomodeum (the future oral cavity) develops as a pit in the midline. The stomodeum is lined with stratified squamous epithelial cells (oral

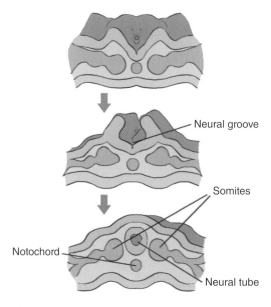

Figure 2.4  Neurulation.

ectoderm) and is separated from the foregut by a buccopharyngeal membrane. This membrane eventually ruptures to establish a connection from the oral cavity to the foregut.

Below the stomodeum, five bars develop from the fourth to seventh prenatal weeks. They develop due to mesoderm thickening and form in the shape of five bars, dorsoventrally to the foregut wall. These are the pharyngeal or branchial arches (Figure 2.5). Only the first two pharyngeal arches have specific names: the mandibular and the hyoid, respectively. Each pharyngeal arch contains muscles, cartilage and blood supply (Table 2.1). The aortic arch blood vessel, leading from the heart to the brain, is crucial to craniofacial development, as it runs through all pharyngeal arches. Pharyngeal pouches separate these bars and give rise to specific structures (Figure 2.6). Ectoderm covers the exterior portion of each arch. The second to fifth arches grow together and create a smooth outer surface. However, the fifth arch disappears soon after development.

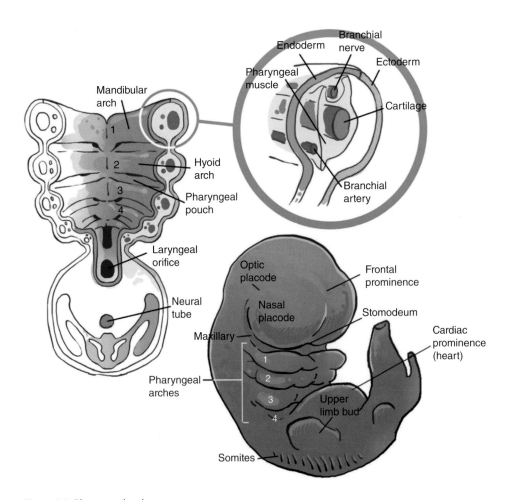

**Figure 2.5** Pharyngeal arches.

Table 2.1  The muscles, cartilages, derivatives and blood supply to the pharyngeal arches.

| Pharyngeal Arch | Blood Supply[a] | Muscles | Cartilage | Derivatives |
|---|---|---|---|---|
| I Mandibular | V Trigeminal | Masticatory:<br>  Masseter<br>  Lateral pterygoid<br>  Medial pterygoid<br>  Temporalis | Meckel's | Mandibular process:<br>  Mandible<br>  Malleus<br>  Incus<br>  Sphenomandibular ligament<br><br>Maxillary process:<br>  Maxilla<br>  Zygoma<br>  Zygomatic process of temporal bone<br><br>Muscles of mastication |
| II Hyoid | VII Facial | Posterior belly of digastric muscle<br>Stapedius<br>Stylohyoid<br><br>Facial expression:<br>  Frontalis<br>  Orbicularis oris<br>  Orbicularis oculi<br>  Zygomaticus<br>  Buccinator<br>  Platysma | Reichart's | Facial muscles<br>Stapes<br>Styloid process of temporal bone<br>Lesser horn<br>Superior body of hyoid bone<br>Stylohyoid ligament |
| III | Glossopharyngeal | Stylopharyngeus | Inferior hyoid | Inferior body of hyoid bone |
| IV | X Vagus | Intrinsic muscles of larynx<br>Cricothyroid<br>Constrictors of pharynx | Laryngeal | Laryngeal cartilages |

[a] Cranial nerve.

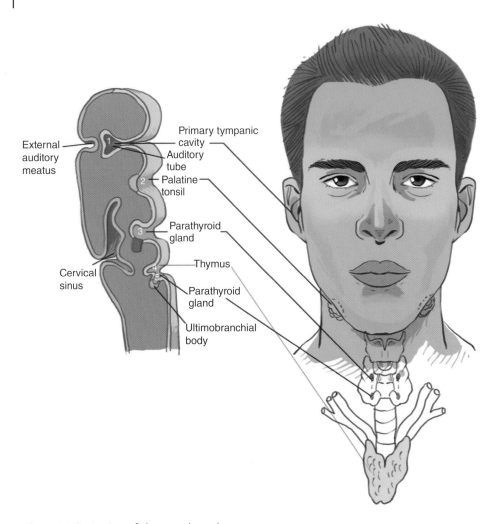

External auditory meatus

Primary tympanic cavity

Auditory tube

Palatine tonsil

Parathyroid gland

Thymus

Cervical sinus

Parathyroid gland

Ultimobranchial body

**Figure 2.6** Derivatives of pharyngeal pouches.

During this phase of embryonic development, the craniofacial growth initiates. The growth of the face relies on the initial cartilage formed, which is known as the primary cartilage. The chondrocranium is the term used for the primitive cartilaginous skeletal structures. The floor of the skull is composed of basicranium, known as the cranial base postnatal. Basicranium derives from the mesenchyme and develops during the fourth prenatal week. During early development, a series of cartilaginous tissues begin the cranial base development. These tissues are mainly composed of chondrocranium.

Towards the end of the second prenatal period, the chondrocranium undergoes ossification (new bone formation). Once the primitive structures are established, the face begins to develop downwards and forwards by the fifth prenatal week. During this phase of development, the embryo attains a curved form and grows dramatically in size, and structured organ systems are evident.

The limbs and organ systems continue to grow by the eighth week as the embryo develops human characteristics. Upon completion of the embryonic period, the third prenatal phase begins; this period is termed the fetal phase.

The embryo is termed a fetus from the ninth prenatal week until birth (Figure 2.7). At this stage, the fetus gains human characteristics. Organs begin to function and established connections between the organs and the systems become obvious. As growth continues, dramatic increase in size and weight is noticeable due to continuing tissue differentiation.

## Craniofacial Postnatal Development

A basic understanding of craniofacial growth is essential for oral health therapists, dental hygienists and dental therapists. Referrals for early detection of some abnormal craniofacial growth can eliminate the need for complex treatment after maturity with early orthodontic intervention (discussed in Chapter 3). A brief summary of several aspects of craniofacial growth is given in this chapter.

The skull consists of two parts known as the neurocranium and the viscerocranium (also called the splanocranium; Figure 2.8).

- Neurocranium: encases the brain – the growth of the cranium relies on the cranial vault (the internal neurocranium space for the brain) and the cranial base (floor of the skull).
- Viscerocranium: the facial portion of the skull – the maxillary and the mandibular growth greatly contribute to the development of the viscerocranium.

### Growth Mechanisms

The human body consists of several growth centres that regulate, control and monitor overall growth of the bones throughout the body. Bone formation (also known as ossification) is dependent upon two major mechanisms: endochondral ossification and intramembranous ossification.

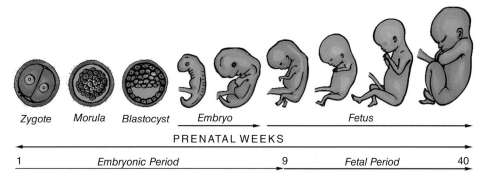

Figure 2.7 Embryo to fetal growth.

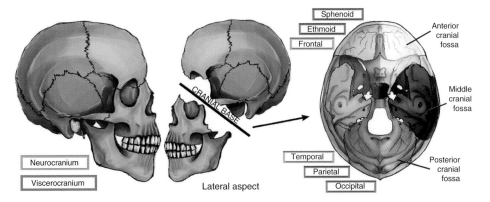

Figure 2.8 Neurocranium and viscerocranium. The cranial base is composed of three hollow depressions called fossae. It consists of several nerve openings for blood supply to the neurocranium.

- Endochondral ossification
  This process is conversion of cartilage into bone. Long bones in the body develop from endochondral ossification. The cranial base and the mandibular condyle contain endochondral bones.
- Intramembranous ossification
  Intramembranous ossification regulates flat bone development. Osseous tissue formation initiates from mesenchymal connective tissue through intramembranous ossification. The cranial vault, maxilla and body of the mandible consist of intramembranous bones.
- Remodelling and displacement
  Another growth mechanism is remodelling, involving bone deposition (new bone laid by osteoblasts) and resorption (mature bone loss by osteoclasts). As a bony structure undergoes remodelling, its position alters and this is known as drift. During early development, several bony plates fuse and form junctions known as sutures. Sutures are fibrous joints also known as syndesmoses. These joints form dense connective tissue regions called fontanelles when they meet and these areas ossify at variable times postnatally.
  The movement of the bone as a unit is called displacement. There are two types of bone displacement:

1) Primary displacement: is when the bone shifts due to its own growth.
2) Secondary displacement: occurs when the bone shifts due to growth of an adjacent bone.

- Synchondrosis

  The cranial vault consists of intramembranous bones. Its enlargement occurs due to growth at the sutures and remodelling as the developing brain expands. The cranial base consists of endochondral bones and its growth occurs within the growth centres at synchondroses (cartilaginous joints between bones). Four different types of synchondroses are significant to the cranial base, as the facial skeletal pattern and the length of the cranial base relies on the growth at these sites:

1) spheno-occipital
2) sphenoethmoidal
3) intersphenoid
4) interoccipital.

### The Neonatal Skull Compared With the Adult Skull

A higher ratio of neurocranium to viscerocranium is obvious in a neonatal skull (Figure 2.9). This dominance is due to the advanced growth of the brain at birth. Thus, the width of viscerocranium is greater than its height in a neonatal skull. The viscero-cranium continues to grow and a substantial increase in the facial height is apparent in an adult skull. This increase in the facial height relies greatly on the development of the upper and lower jaws. The postnatal rate of growth is reduced during the prepubertal stages. However, a very high rate of growth is evident during the initial pubertal period, which is known as the growth spurt, reflecting this rapid growth. This increased rate slows down as the pubertal stage terminates. On average, girls reach the growth spurt by 12 years of age and boys at around 14 years of age; this stage lasts for about two years.

The skull is a complex structure developed from mesenchymal connective tissue that surrounds the developing brain. Growth is particularly important in orthodontics, as the impact of growth is considered in diagnosis and treatment planning. Orthodontists always observe how growth has contributed to malocclusion or facial deformities in all patients and determine how several growth patterns can influence or favour the tenta-tive treatment options in growing patients.

### Mandibular Growth

As mentioned previously, the growth and development of the viscerocranium depends on the mandibular and nasomaxillary growth (Figure 2.10). The first pharyngeal arch cartilage (Meckel's cartilage) supports the primitive mandible. During early mandibular development, intramembranous ossification spreads anteriorly and posteriorly. This type of ossification forms the mandibular symphysis, a portion of the body of the

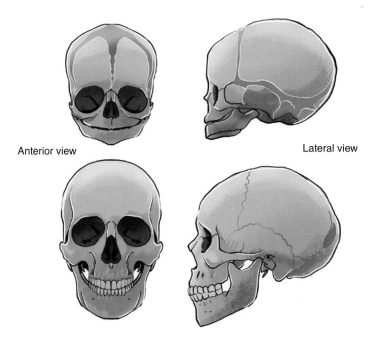

Anterior view          Lateral view

Figure 2.9 The infant skull compared with the adult skull.

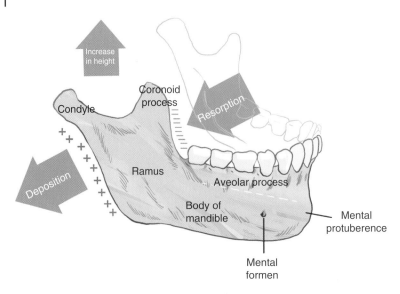

Figure 2.10 Mandibular growth. Generally, growth at the condyle takes place in two directions: upwards and backwards. The mandible displaces forwards and downwards.

mandible and a part of the ramus. The neonate mandible consists of two halves, which unite at the midline by the first postnatal year.

The long-term growth of the mandible is through endochondral ossification, resulting in downward and forward displacement. Remodelling of the mandible greatly contributes to the increase in width of the mandible during maturation. Deposition takes place posterior to the ramus as resorption occurs anteriorly to the ramus, thus making the ramus grow away from the chin.

The mandibular condyle is an articulating surface; a cartilage therefore covers the peripheral portion of the condyle. The growth cartilage within the condyle allows endochondral ossification to take place. The condylar process, the coronoid process and the mental process consist of endochondral bones. Condylar growth increases the height of the ramus. The alveolar process, supported by the body of the mandible, greatly contributes to an increase in height of the corpus (the body of the mandible). On average, the growth of the mandible ceases at around 17 years in girls and 19 years in boys.

### Maxillary Growth

Early maxillary development is a consequence of direct bone deposition into connective tissue, as there are no precursor cartilages (Figure 2.11). The maxilla matures by intramembranous ossification and by bone deposition at the sutures and surface remodelling.

The growth centre of the maxilla lies above the canine enamel organ. Backward growth of the ossified tissues proceeds towards the zygomatic bone. When the tissue growth spreads upwards and forwards, it will give rise to the frontal process of the maxilla and the incisor regions, respectively. The downward bone deposition will become the maxillary alveolar plate, which contributes to an increase in height of the maxilla. On average, the growth of the maxilla terminates by about 15 years of age in girls and 17 years in boys. The maxillary periosteal remodelling masks the rotational growth effect

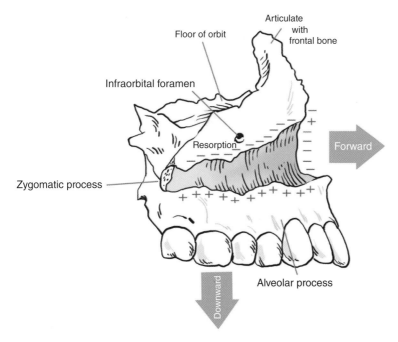

Figure 2.11 Maxillary growth.

of the upper jaw. The maxilla displaces downwards and forwards due to both primary and secondary displacement.

- During primary displacement: the growth at the tuberosity region can push the maxilla against the cranial base and results in the downward and forward shift.
- During secondary displacement: the maxilla moves downward and forward due to the cranial base growth.

As a result of remodelling, bone deposition occurs in the inferior region of the palate as resorption takes place in the superior region. The downward growth of the maxilla also relies on:

- the inferior drift of the hard palate
- eruption of the maxillary teeth
- the development of the alveolar process.

### Growth Rotation

The curved direction of the growth results in a rotational effect, which was described by Solow and Houston in 1988. This effect is minimal in the maxilla and substantial in the mandible, and is apparent on the vertical plane. The growth of several structures compromises the direction of growth. Clinically, growth rotation is assessed by the anterior facial height and the mandibular plane. If the growth of the mandibular condyle is greater than the vertical growth of the molar regions, the mandible rotates counter-clockwise. This results in a lower placement of the mandible, with a patent forward rotation. Patients present with decreased anterior facial heights, flattening of the

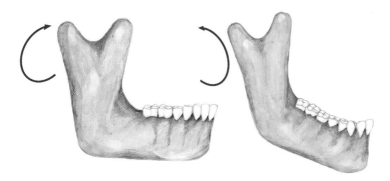

Figure 2.12 Growth rotation. The forward growth presents with a convergent mandibular angle. Backward growth presents with a steep divergent mandibular angle.

mandibular plane and an anterior overbite. As the severity of the forward rotation increases, the anterior overbite becomes deeper.

The sagittal growth of the mandibular condyle results in a backward growth of the mandible as it grows in the direction of its length. The backward growth presents with an increased anterior facial height and a steep mandibular plane angle. This results in an anterior overjet or an anterior open bite in severe cases. This occurs when the condylar growth is less than the vertical growth of the molar region, so the mandible rotates clockwise. Orthodontists always consider the rotational growth effects prior to treatment planning to minimise the precipitated effects from relapse due to further rotational growth during and after treatment.

Forward growth of the mandible results in an upright path of incisor eruption, whereas backward growth rotation generates an anterior path of incisor eruption (Gill, 2008). Late incisor crowding has been associated with mandibular growth rotation for the following reasons:

- Forward mandibular growth: the length of the arch becomes reduced, with incisor becoming more upright, resulting in lower anterior crowding (Figure 2.12).
- Backward mandibular growth: as the mandible rotates backwards, the lower incisors are pushed against the lower lip, precipitating the incisors to become more upright, thus leading to lower anterior crowding (Figure 2.13).

## Tooth Development

### Initial development

Odontogenesis or tooth development begins at the sixth prenatal week (Figure 2.14). The oral epithelium is lined by stratified, squamous epithelial cells known as the oral ectoderm. The overlaying connective tissues (derived from neural crest cells) instruct the oral ectoderm to initiate tooth development. A series of interactions between the epithelium and the ectomesenchymal cells result in tooth formation and development. A basement membrane separates the ectomesenchymal cells from the oral epithelium (Figure 2.15). A primary epithelial band proliferates from the surface of the oral ectoderm

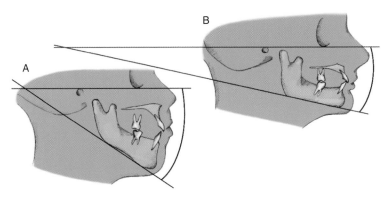

Figure 2.13 Growth rotation: A) Increased facial height is evident with backward growth rotation. B) Reduced facial height is seen in forward growth rotation.

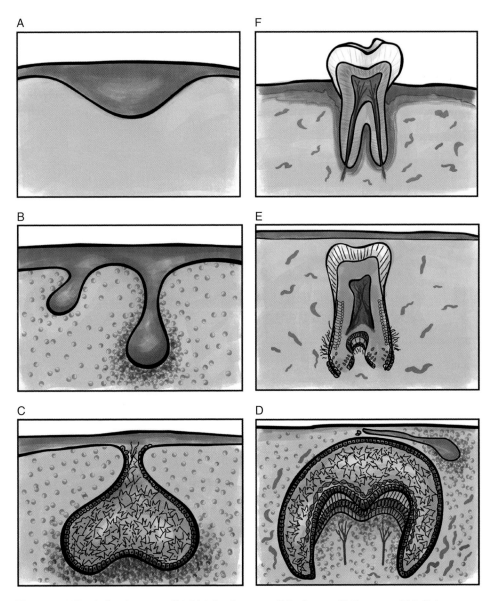

Figure 2.14 Tooth development: A) Initial development. B) Bud stage. C) Cap stage. D) Bell stage. E) Root formation. F) Eruption.

and resembles a horseshoe structure. This band determines the position of the upper and lower arches. The primary epithelial band gives rise to two structures:

1) The vestibular lamina is an invagination that forms the future oral vestibules to separate the cheeks and lip.
2) The dental lamina gives rise to the teeth.

### Bud Stage

The dental lamina pushes through the mesenchyme in the form of ten swellings in each arch. The term given to these localised protuberances is the tooth bud (Figure 2.16). These initial bulges develop into deciduous teeth. By the fifth prenatal week, more tooth buds develop from the dental lamina extensions to give rise to the permanent successors. This leading edge of the dental lamina is called the successional lamina. However, the term successional lamina is only given to the extensions of the 20 primary teeth buds. The permanent molars develop from the general lamina. At this stage, the crown morphology is determined by the tooth bud. Defects during this stage of tooth development can lead to absence of tooth buds or extra tooth bud formation, causing hypodontia (missing teeth) or hyperdontia (extra teeth), respectively.

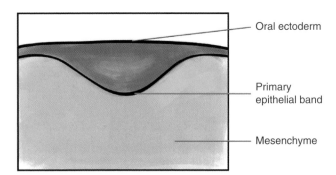

Figure 2.15 Initial tooth development.

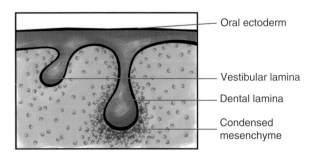

Figure 2.16 Bud stage.

## Cap Stage

The mesenchymal cells surrounding the dental lamina begin to condense (Figure 2.17). This compression results in a depression of the peripheral surface of the tooth bud. Dental papillae form as the condensed mesenchyme travels deeper into the dental lamina concavity. This will give rise to the dental pulp. The epithelial cells become the enamel organ. These papillae will give rise to the enamel and the dentine through several interactions and differentiations in the next stage of development. Outer enamel epithelial cells cover the outer layer of the enamel organ in a single layer. These cells are cuboidal in shape. A single layer of inner enamel epithelial cells covers the inner concavity of the enamel organ. These cells are columnar in shape. Stellate reticulum are star shaped cells that separates the outer and inner enamel epithelium.

Localised areas on the surface of the inner enamel epithelium coalesce to form enamel knots. These enamel knots lengthen towards the outer enamel epithelium in the form of strands called the enamel cords. These two structures have a major role in cusp position and disappear upon mineralisation.

## Bell Stage

The bell stage is vital as the enamel organ cultivates, because of two major events of morphodifferentiation and histodifferentiation (Figure 2.18). During morphodifferentiation, the shape of the tooth is determined. Through histodifferentiation, several cell

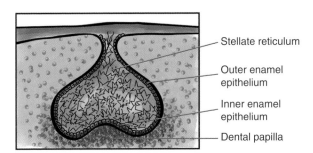

Stellate reticulum

Outer enamel epithelium

Inner enamel epithelium

Dental papilla

**Figure 2.17** Cap stage.

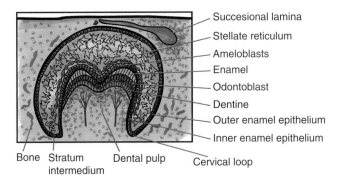

Succesional lamina
Stellate reticulum
Ameloblasts
Enamel
Odontoblast
Dentine
Outer enamel epithelium
Inner enamel epithelium

Bone   Stratum         Dental pulp      Cervical loop
       intermedium

**Figure 2.18** Bell stage.

interactions and differentiations occur for definite structures to develop. The enamel organ resembles a bell at this stage, as the cells get prepared for enamel and dentine formation. Adjacent to the inner enamel epithelium lies a layer of cells called the stratum intermedium. These cells are essential in enamel formation.

A dense fibrous mesodermal layer, known as the dental follicle or dental sac, surrounds the epithelial portion of the enamel organ. The periodontal ligaments, cementum and the alveolar bone proper are dental follicle derivatives. The inner enamel epithelium and outer enamel epithelium meet to form the cervical loop. The enamel organ gradually detaches from the epithelium by this stage. The residuals of the dental lamina are called the rests of Serres. The differentiation and mineralisation of tissues in the crown begin from the incisal edge and progress apically. A series of inductive interactions regulate the bell stage.

The bell stage inductive interactions are:

- The inner enamel epithelium interacts with the undifferentiated mesenchymal cells in the dental papilla. The result of this interaction leads to formation of odontoblasts. These cells then become columnar and elongated to give rise to a mineralised organic matrix called predentin. It takes 24 hours for dentine to develop as predentin calcifies. Layers of dentine lay in increments at the future dentinoenamel junction. The dental pulp develops as dentine covers the entire surrounding of the dental papilla. During this stage, the dental pulp generates a fine vascular network associated with the odontoblastic layer. Dentinal tubules maintain the elongating process of odontoblasts. This process of dentine formation is called dentinogenesis.
- During amelogenesis, the inner enamel epithelial cells differentiate upon dentine deposition at the site of the future dentinoenamel junction and become secretory ameloblasts. Nutrition supply to ameloblasts infiltrates via the stellate reticulum from the outer enamel epithelium. Blood is supplied through an organised network of capillaries. Once the inner enamel epithelium differentiates into ameloblasts, enamel deposits in increments at the site and dentinoenamel junction is marked.

Amelogenin is a protein that mineralises the matrix. The matured enamel protein is termed enamelin. The enamel undergoes maturation as it loses all water and organic material, because of the high mineral content. The presence of excessive fluoride during this phase of development of the permanent dentition leads to interference of water and organic material loss. Nevertheless, fluorosis occurs and white opaque patches will be present on the enamel surface after eruption.

Upon completion of mineralisation and maturation, the ameloblasts shorten to meet the stratum intermedium and the outer enamel epithelium; this is known as reduced enamel epithelium, covering the enamel surface until eruption.

Congenital abnormalities during this phase of tooth development may result in enamel or dentine defects such as denetinogenesis imperfecta or amelogenesis imperfecta. Dentinogenesis imperfecta makes the dentine opalescent and the enamel prone to breakage, wear and loss from weakness. Amelogenesis imperfecta is an enamel protein malfunction causing abnormal enamel formation, affecting the shape and colour of the enamel.

## Root Formation

Once the crown development is completed, the cells begin to migrate apically until they reach the future cementoenamel junction. The outer and inner enamel epithelium meet, forming an epithelial root sheath, also known as Hertwig's root sheath. This structure determines the length, thickness and number of roots. The curved and bent edge of the epithelial root sheath is called epithelial diaphragm.

Dentine formation initiates root formation (Figure 2.19). The inner enamel epithelium (ameloblasts) induces the odontoblast of the dental papilla to differentiate into dentine. The root sheath begins to break down on the surface of the developing root, exposing the dentine to the surrounding dental follicles. Interaction between dentine and the dental follicles leads to the formation of cementoblasts, which lay cementum in increments. Residuals of the root sheath are known as epithelial cell rests of Malassez. The dental follicle surrounding the root also differentiates into osteoblasts and fibroblasts to give rise to alveolar bone and periodontal ligaments, respectively. As root dentinogenesis continues, the root lengthens and initiates tooth eruption and creates space apically to allow sufficient root growth.

## Eruption

Table 2.2 shows the approximate dates of eruption for human teeth. There are several studies and debatable theories regarding tooth eruption. However, three phases can summarise tooth eruption:

1) The pre-eruptive phase: prior to eruption and during early development, when the crown is covered by an overlaying mucosa.
2) Prefunctional phase: when the tooth pushes through the mucosa by contacting the oral epithelium as the reduced enamel epithelium disintegrates the connective tissue.
3) Functional phase: when the tooth is in occlusion and functioning.

It is essential for all dental practitioners to recognise eruption delays or abnormalities in patients and refer to orthodontists as needed.

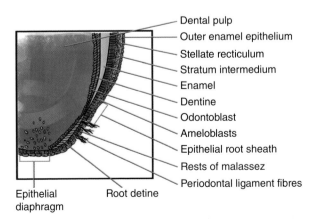

Epithelial diaphragm  Root detine

Dental pulp
Outer enamel epithelium
Stellate recticulum
Stratum intermedium
Enamel
Dentine
Odontoblast
Ameloblasts
Epithelial root sheath
Rests of malassez
Periodontal ligament fibres

**Figure 2.19** Root formation.

Table 2.2 Tooth eruption dates.

| Dentition | Position | Eruption dates |
| --- | --- | --- |
| Central incisors | Upper primary | 6–10 months |
| | Lower primary | 5–8 months |
| | Permanent upper | 7–8 years |
| | Permanent lower | 6–7 years |
| Lateral incisors | Upper primary | 8–12 months |
| | Lower primary | 7–10 months |
| | Permanent upper | 8–9 years |
| | Permanent lower | 7–8 years |
| Canines | Upper and lower primary | 16–20 months |
| | Permanent upper | 11–12 years |
| | Permanent lower | 9–11 years |
| Premolars: | | |
| First | Permanent upper | 10–11 years |
| | Permanent lower | 10–12 years |
| Second | Permanent upper | 10–12 years |
| | Permanent lower | 11–13 years |
| Molars: | | |
| First | Primary (upper and lower) | 11–18 months |
| | Permanent (upper and lower) | 6–7 years |
| Second | Primary (upper and lower) | 20–30 months |
| | Permanent (upper and lower) | 12–14 years |
| Third | Permanent (upper and lower) | ≥17 years |

# References

Gill D. S. *Orthodontics at a Glance*. Oxford: Wiley-Blackwell Publishing; 2008.
Solow B, Houston W. Mandibular rotations: concepts and terminology. *Eur J Orthod* 1988; 10(3): 177–179.

# Further Reading

Ahmad, I. Digital dental photography. Part 1: an overview. *Br Dental J*, 2009; 206: 403–407.
Bishara, S. E. *Textbook of Orthodontics*. Philadelphia, PA: W.B. Saunders; 2001.
Brand, R. W., Isselhard, D. E. *Anatomy of Orofacial Structures: A comprehensive approach*. 7th ed. St Louis, MO: Elsevier Mosby.
Chiego, D. J. *Essentials of Oral Histology and Embryology: A clinical approach*. 4th ed. St Louis, MO: Elsevier Mosby; 2014.

Downs, W. B. Analysis of the dentofacial profile. *Angle Orthod*, 1956; 26(4): 191–212.

Foster, T. D. *A Textbook of Orthodontics*. 3rd ed. Oxford: Blackwell Scientific; 1990.

Goose, D. H., Appleton, J. *Human Dentofacial Growth*. Oxford: Pergamon Press; 1982.

Mitchell, L. *An Introduction to Orthodontics*. 3rd ed. Oxford: Oxford University Press; 2007.

Ooë, T. *Human Tooth and Dental Arch Development*. Tokyo: Ishiyaku Publishers; 1981.

Park, J. U., Baik, S. H. Classification of angle class III malocclusion and its treatment modalities. *Int J Adult Orthod*, 2001; 16(1): 19–29.

Proffit, W. R., Fields H. W. Jr, Sarver, D. *Contemporary Orthodontics*. 5th ed. St Louis, MO: Mosby Elsevier; 2012.

Ranly, D. M. *A Synopsis of Craniofacial Growth*. 2nd ed. Norwalk, CT: Appleton & Lange; 1990.

Thesleff, I. Epithelial–mesenchymal signaling regulating tooth morphogenesis. *J Cell Science*, 2003; 116(9): 1647–1648.

Thilander, B. Basic mechanisms in craniofacial growth. *Acta Odontol Scand*, 1995; 53(3): 144–151.

Welbury, R. R., Duggal, M. S., Hosey, M. T. *Paediatric Dentistry*. 4th ed. Oxford: Oxford University Press; 2012.

## Self-Evaluation

1 What is embryogenesis?
   **A** Sperm penetrating through the egg barriers.
   **B** Formation and development of an embryo.
   **C** Multiplication of embryo cells.
   **D** Travelling of the embryo from the fallopian tube to the uterus.

2 How are pharyngeal arches developed?
   **A** Thickening of the mesoderm.
   **B** Derived from the endoderm.
   **C** Developed during gastrulation.
   **D** Thickening of the ectodermal layers.

3 Which pharyngeal arch is responsible for the development of the mandible?
   **A** First pharyngeal arch.
   **B** Second pharyngeal arch.
   **C** Third pharyngeal arch.
   **D** Fourth pharyngeal arch.

4 Which pharyngeal pouch develops into the palatine tonsils?
   **A** First pharyngeal pouch.
   **B** Second pharyngeal pouch.
   **C** Third pharyngeal pouch.
   **D** Fourth pharyngeal pouch.

5  How is flat bone development regulated?
   **A** Intramembranous ossification.
   **B** Remodelling.
   **C** Displacement.
   **D** Intramembranous ossification and displacement.

6  In which directions does the maxilla grow during secondary displacement?
   **A** Upwards and forwards.
   **B** Downwards and forwards.
   **C** Backwards and forwards.
   **D** Backwards and downwards.

7  What is the name given to the facial portion of the skull?
   **A** Viscerocranium.
   **B** Neurocranium.
   **C** Splanocranium.
   **D** A and C.

8  During which stage of tooth development can hyperdontia and hypodontia occur?
   **A** Dentinogenesis.
   **B** Amelogenesis.
   **C** Root formation.
   **D** Bud stage.

9  At what stage of embryonic development does initial tooth development begin?
   **A** 3 weeks in utero.
   **B** 12 weeks in utero.
   **C** 6 weeks in utero.
   **D** 4 weeks in utero.

10  Name the tooth developmental stages in order.
    **A** Cap stage, bell stage, bud stage.
    **B** Bell stage, cap stage, bud stage.
    **C** Bud stage, cap stage, bell stage.
    **D** Bud stage, bell stage, cap stage.

3

# Orthodontic Assessment and Treatment Planning Strategies

This chapter reviews the steps involved in an orthodontic assessment and briefly evaluates the principles of treatment planning. Diagnosis and treatment planning in an orthodontic practice is solely the responsibility of an orthodontist. Oral health therapists and dental hygienists carry out necessary examinations and clinical procedures within their scope of practice under the supervision of an orthodontist. Nevertheless, it is crucial to have a thorough knowledge and understanding of the processes involved in an orthodontic assessment and treatment planning.

This process commences with a patient interview to address the patient's concerns, identifying the issues and developing a list of problems. Patient interviews provide valuable information that is critical in planning for successful treatment outcomes. Accurate analysis of all gathered records, including photographs, radiographs and study models of the teeth, leads to an accurate diagnosis and thus a successful treatment outcome.

Risks and benefits of the chosen treatment plan should be discussed with the patient and parent (if the patient is under the legal age of consent) to gain an informed consent, which is the final stage prior to commencement of the chosen treatment. It is critical that explanations are given in a simple manner with the use of terminology that is easy for parents and patients to understand.

## Data Collection

Gathering an accurate and detailed patient history aids in diagnosis and treatment planning. Comprehensive records are extremely valuable as they reveal vital information regarding the general health, oral health and social and family history of the patient. During the patient and parent interview, several factors may be revealed that could compromise the treatment plan. Accurate and thorough data collection and history taking are therefore extremely important.

Clinicians must obtain a medical and dental history at initial appointments, and should review the information at subsequent visits, and update this information every six months for better patient management.

The initial appointments in an orthodontic practice are dedicated to patient interviews and consultations. This allows the dental team to get to know the patient better, to gain a better understanding of their attitude and assess their level of understanding of their orthodontic condition. These interviews are essential for better patient

*Orthodontics for Dental Hygienists and Dental Therapists*, First Edition. Tina Raked.
© 2018 John Wiley & Sons Ltd. Published 2018 by John Wiley & Sons Ltd.
Companion website: www.wiley.com/go/raked/orthodontics_dental_hygienists

management, as the lifestyle of the patient is considered when treatment planning to ensure that they benefit from their orthodontic treatment.

### Medical History

The objective behind taking a detailed medical history is to provide a beneficial orthodontic treatment without the patient suffering from any medical complications and to avoid medical emergencies. This can be achieved by considering the medical contraindications when treatment planning (examples of these contraindications and modified treatment planning are summarised in Table 3.1). Growth is another aspect that requires specific attention as it facilitates orthodontic treatment. Beyond the growth spurt peak, orthodontists may need to alter the treatment plan to accommodate for changes in the facial structures to prevent the treatment outcome being compromised. Box 3.1 highlights some areas covered in a medical history form. The growth assessment and the record of onset of puberty is essential in children and young adults.

### Dental History

The dental history provides valuable information regarding the motivation and cooperation of the patient in a dental setting. Gaining a better understanding of previous dental treatments and oral hygiene habits determines the level of motivation. Attending regular dental check-ups is a good indication that the patient will comply with their orthodontic appointments as well. The dental history must be thorough, including details of any previous treatments, attitude and behaviour towards previous treatments and records of any dental trauma. One of the main contraindications of orthodontic treatment is poor oral hygiene, as the patient will be at high risk of caries and periodontal disease. It is important to record the oral hygiene regimen, such as the type of toothbrush and toothpaste used, as well as the technique and frequency of brushing. Box 3.2 highlights some areas covered in a dental history form.

### Patient Concerns

Chief complaints reveal the patient's perception of their concern, whether it be aesthetics or functional. This may or may not be the same reason as the initial referral by other colleagues. Addressing the chief complaint is key to reaching a successful treatment outcome. It is vital for practitioners to understand the patient's concern and it is just as critical to ensure that the patient understands their orthodontic problem and in what ways it can be treated. For example, a patient might request treatment in the upper jaw because of excessive protrusion, yet the underlying problem may indicate a mandible that is retrusive and requires a more complicated treatment than the patient anticipated. Before treatment starts, the patient needs to have a thorough understanding of their functional and aesthetic orthodontic problem and accept the procedures and steps involved in their chosen treatment. Addressing the chief complaint also increases patient compliance.

### Aetiology of Malocclusion

Investigating the cause of any underlying dental discrepancy is necessary. If the aetiology is unknown, a successful treatment outcome may not be guaranteed. Hereditary factors or environmental factors may contribute to the cause of the malocclusion. Eliminating

Table 3.1 Medical conditions and orthodontic implications for treatment.

| Medical Alert | Concerns | Modifications for Orthodontic Treatment |
|---|---|---|
| Infective endocarditis | Risk of bacteraemia in the inner tissues of the heart causing infection and inflammation. | Separators, impressions and surgical tooth exposures may require antibiotic prophylaxis.<br>Bonding is a better option than banding.<br>Always maintain oral hygiene and monitor plaque control.<br>Avoid mucosal cuts during rewire replacements.<br>Always confirm treatment with patient's cardiologist or physician. |
| Hypertension | High blood pressure can put the patient at risk of cardiovascular disease, renal failure and stroke. The major concern is gingival hyperplasia due to calcium channel blockers. Therefore, any signs of gingival overgrowth requires immediate attention. | To reduce stress levels, the appointments should be kept to less than one hour.<br>Regular oral hygiene advice is necessary to ensure that plaque control is achieved.<br>If calcium channel blockers cause gingival hyperplasia, refer to physician for new prescriptions.<br>Delay treatment for uncontrolled hypertension until the physician confirms the condition is under control. |
| Diabetes | Hyperglycaemia causes delayed healing and patients are at higher risk of periodontal disease. This is due to reduced leucocyte function, low collagen metabolism and reduced polymorphonuclear leucocyte.<br>Periodic periodontal assessment is necessary in patients with both type I (insulin dependent) and type II (insulin resistant) diabetes. | Owing to periodontal breakdown, avoid treatment in patients with uncontrolled diabetes. Always confirm with the physician before starting treatment.<br>Reduce local factors such as calculus by stressing the importance of immaculate oral hygiene.<br>Appointments are best to be scheduled after breakfast. |

(Continued)

Table 3.1 (Continued)

| Medical Alert | Concerns | Modifications for Orthodontic Treatment |
|---|---|---|
| Epilepsy | Gingival hypertrophy is associated with anticonvulsants causing red, swollen and sore gums. Studies have shown high doses of antiepileptic medications during early growth and development can affect the child's skull development, position of teeth and periodontal structures.<br><br>Other oral findings associated with antiepileptic medication include hypercementosis, root shortenings, gingival bleeding, xerostomia, ulceration and delayed eruption.<br><br>It is essential to record history of seizures, related traumas and details of medication.<br><br>Patients are also at risk of inhaling or swallowing fragments of appliances during seizures; nevertheless, it is important to advise patients and parents/carers to seek medical advice immediately | Gingival contouring may be needed prior to bracket positioning in cases of severe gingival hypertrophy.<br><br>Minimize stress levels during treatment.<br><br>Cease procedure immediately if seizure occurs during treatment, retrieve all instruments from the mouth and lower the chair in a supine position as low as possible.<br><br>If the seizure does not cease within a few minutes, seek help immediately. |
| Pregnancy | There are generally no contraindications associated with pregnancy. However, increased levels of progesterone and estrogen can cause an exaggerated response to plaque. It is essential to assess periodontal health frequently. | Monitor oral health and review oral hygiene each visit.<br><br>Keep appointments short and avoid x-rays. |
| Thyroid disorders | The hormones produced by the thyroid gland are responsible for growth, development and metabolism in the body. Common oral findings in hypothyroidism include delayed wound healing, macroglossia, delayed eruption and periodontal disease. Patients with hyperthyroidism can suffer from stress and anxiety. | Reduce stress levels throughout treatment and avoid the use of adrenaline.<br><br>Cease treatment in the case of thyrotoxic crisis.<br><br>Ensure that the patient visits their physician regularly.<br><br>A thyroid collar is critical for taking radiographs for protection against radiation. |
| Infectious diseases | The major concern for patients with infectious diseases such as hepatitis and HIV would be maintaining good oral hygiene and high standard infection control as per guidelines. | Follow universal precaution guidelines.<br><br>Good oral hygiene.<br><br>Check treatment with haematologist for any medical contraindications. |

**Box 3.1  Some Areas Covered in a Medical History Form**

- Patient details (name, age, address, number).
- Details of general practitioner.
- Growth assessment: birth weight, current weight, height, onset of puberty.
- *For female adolescents only*: Has menarche (first period) occurred?
- Stomach ulcer or hyperacidity.
- Cancer or been treated for a tumour.
- Diabetes.
- Immune system conditions.
- Kidney conditions.
- Endocrine or thyroid conditions.
- Arthritic conditions.
- Mental or behavioural conditions.
- Ear, eye, throat, nose or speech conditions.
- Tonsil or adenoid conditions.
- Loss of weight or poor appetite.
- Fainting, seizures or epilepsy.
- Anaemia or bleeding disorder.
- AIDS or HIV positive.
- Hepatitis.
- High or low blood pressure.
- History of asthma, hay fever, sinus or hives.
- Cardiovascular conditions (heart attack, angina, coronary insufficiency, arteriosclerosis, stroke, inborn heart defects or rheumatic heart).
- Polio, mononucleosis, tuberculosis, pneumonia.
- Current allergies or drug reactions.
- Medication the patient is currently taking (prescription/non-prescription/supplements).
- Past surgical procedures.

**Box 3.2  Some Areas Covered in a Dental History Form**

- Permanent or 'extra' teeth removed.
- Chipped or otherwise damaged teeth or missing fillings.
- Teeth sensitive to heat or cold.
- Non-vital teeth or root canal treated.
- Jaw fractures, cysts or mouth infections.
- Gum problems, such as bleeding gums.
- Has patient ever had periodontal (gum) treatment?
- Food impaction between teeth.
- Thumb or finger sucking habit.
- History of speech problems.
- Snoring or difficulty in breathing.
- Grinding, jaw clenching or clicking.
- Any pain or soreness in the muscles of the face or around the jaw.
- Difficulty in chewing or jaw opening.
- Any wisdom teeth problems.
- Any relatives with similar tooth or jaw conditions.
- Has patient had any serious trouble with previous dental treatment?
- Has the patient had prior orthodontic treatment?
- Main concern/s about patient's teeth.

environmental causes will allow better interception and enhances treatment stability. For example, if a child presents with normal craniofacial growth and an anterior open bite caused by a thumb sucking habit, it is critical to plan habit breakers as part of the treatment to cease the habit and to reduce the chances of relapse upon completion of treatment. The aetiology of malocclusion is multifactorial in nature and may be due to skeletal discrepancies, dentoalveolar issues and habits. Skeletal discrepancies can be the most difficult to treat because of their widespread effect and it may require a combination of orthodontic treatment and orthopaedic appliances or surgical correction. Dentoalveolar factors may have localised effects on the occlusion. Examples include anomalies in the position of teeth, the number of teeth, eruption patterns, crowding, spacing or pathological abnormalities such as cysts and odontogenic tumours.

## Clinical Examination

The clinical dental examination is an essential part of dentistry and guides every treatment plan. A thorough orthodontic examination begins with a systematic extra- and intraoral examination.

### Extraoral Examination

The findings of a thorough extraoral examination greatly aids in treatment planning. The extraoral examination includes a general assessment of the patient's awareness, posture, temporomandibular joint, head, neck, skeletal pattern and soft tissues. It is important to observe the patient at rest and in function, without their awareness. This approach increases the accuracy of the assessment. The extraoral examination commences in the waiting room or consultation room by observing:

- posture
- awareness
- compliance
- level of comprehension and communication.

### Facial Type and Skeletal Pattern

A valuable aspect of the extraoral examination is identifying the facial type (Figure 3.1) and skeletal pattern (Figure 3.2). The patient must be in a neutral position, sitting upright or standing, looking at a distant object straight ahead. Ensure that the Frankfort plane is horizontal and parallel to the floor by imagining a line from the upper border of the external auditory meatus to the lower border of the orbit (McDonald, 1998). It is important to ensure that the teeth are in centric relation and biting in maximum interdigitation, as these factors affect the accuracy of the examination. Some patients tend to posture the mandible forward and a false diagnosis can be recorded. The frontal view allows an evaluation of the facial type. The sagittal view allows an assessment of the skeletal pattern. On the lateral profile of the patient imagine two lines:

1) From the bridge of the nose to the base of the upper lip.
2) Extending from the base of the upper lip to the base of the chin.

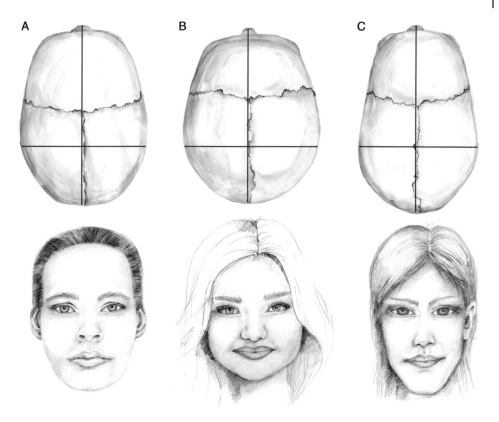

**Figure 3.1** Facial types. A) Mesofacial: well-balanced facial features with average cranial width. B) Brachyfacial: square-shaped faces with a prominent chin and a broad forehead, giving the appearance of a short, wide face. C) Dolichofacial: long narrow face with a small cranial width.

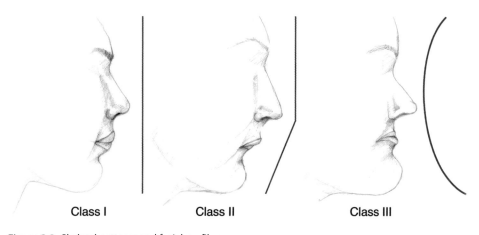

Class I          Class II          Class III

**Figure 3.2** Skeletal patterns and facial profiles.

These lines are an indication of the facial profile and a straight line is considered to be the norm (class I). In a skeletal class II, a convex profile is evident, owing to prominence of the maxilla. In a skeletal class III, concavity in the profile is evident, owing to prominence of the mandible.

Facial appearance is evaluated in three planes of space: anteroposterior, vertical and transverse.

*Anteroposterior*  This is the assessment of the relative position of the maxilla and the mandible. It is classified as:

- Class I skeletal pattern: the mandible is about 2–3 mm posterior to the maxilla. The patient presents with a straight profile, known as a mesognathic profile. The harmony between the maxilla and the mandible creates this straight profile.
- Class II skeletal pattern: the mandible is too far posterior in relation to the maxilla. The patient presents with a convex profile, known as a retrognathic profile. This discrepancy may be due to a protrusive maxilla or a retrusive mandible:
  - Protrusive maxilla: the mandible is in a normal position but the maxilla is positioned too far forward.
  - Retrusive mandible: the maxilla is in the normal position but the mandible is positioned too far posterior in relation to the maxilla.
- Class III skeletal pattern: the mandible is positioned anterior to the maxilla. The patient presents with a concave profile, known as a prognathic profile due to the overgrowth of the mandible.

The dental base supports the alveolar process without the presence of a distinct barrier. Protrusion of both maxillary and mandibular alveolar processes is known as a bimaxillary protrusion (Figure 3.3). This protrusion of the alveolar process in the upper and lower arches can occur concomitantly with class I, class II or class III skeletal bases. Clinically, this is presented by protrusive and everted lips that are separated at rest; hence, incompetent lips. If both the upper and lower alveolar processes are retruded regardless of the skeletal base characteristics, this is termed bimaxillary retrusion.

*Vertical*  Assessment of the lower facial height (Figure 3.4) provides a good indication of any vertical discrepancies:

- Upper third: the forehead.
- Middle third: supraorbital ridge to the base of the nose.
- Lower third: base of the nose to the base of the chin. The lower portion is further classified as:
  - The lower one-third is from the base of the nose to the base of the upper lip.
  - The lower two-thirds consists of the lower lip and chin.

The height of the middle third should equal to height of the lower third. An increase lower facial height is commonly seen in patients with a class III skeletal base owing to the prominence of the chin. A decreased lower facial height is seen in patients with class II skeletal base with a retrusive mandible.

*Transverse*  A mild asymmetry can be considered to be normal. However, any asymmetry must be noted clearly as part of the extra oral examination. This may be due to discrepancies in the transverse sizes of the maxilla and/or the mandible.

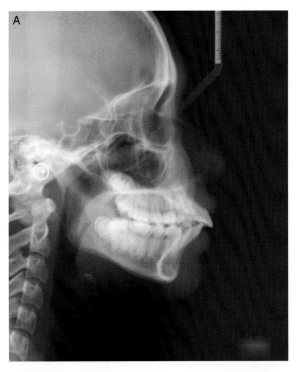

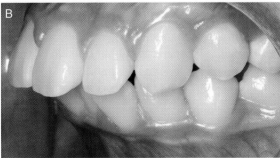

Figure 3.3 A) The lateral cephalometric radiograph confirms the bimaxillary protrusion of the anterior segment. B) Intraoral photograph shows the protruded upper and lower incisors.

**Assessment of Lymph Nodes and the Temporomandibular Joint**
The head and neck regions are examined for any alerts that may indicate an underlying condition, which may require specific attention prior to starting the treatment. The head and neck must be palpated to ensure that the lymph nodes are of normal size and no abnormalities can be detected.

The temporomandibular joint and the surrounding muscles must be checked for anomalies such as tenderness, crepitus (clicking sound that occurs due to friction between cartilage and bone) and deviations that can affect the orthodontist's therapeutic approach and appliance design. If the patient presents with one or more signs of irregularities, a referral to an oral maxillofacial surgeon may be indicated for further investigations.

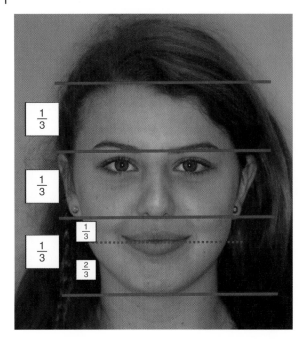

Figure 3.4 Facial height.

### Soft Tissue Analysis

This part of the examination is most effectively and accurately achieved by assessing the patient in function and at rest, without their awareness. It is important to note the following as part of the soft tissue analysis:

- Lip morphology: fullness, tone and form of the lips.
- Lip competency and anterior oral seal: determine how well the upper and lower lips can meet without muscular effort. Lip incompetency may be due to a bimaxillary protrusion, short resting lip length, increased lower anterior face height or protruded upper incisors due to a severe class II. If the lips are incompetent, a normal anterior oral seal will not be achieved.
- Smile framework: the dental midline will set a starting point for achieving an aesthetically pleasing smile. Ideally, the dental midline needs to be parallel and in the same direction as the facial midline. The degree of incisor display and smile symmetry are important aesthetic parameters.
  - The lip line: the position of the upper lip is pivotal to the degree of upper incisor display. This exposure of the height of the incisors is called the lip line. Reduced incisor display may be an indication of aging. The lip line must reach the gingival margin, displaying upper incisal edges and the interdental gingiva. A 'gummy smile' is the term given to a higher than average lip line, which exposes excessive gingiva.
  - The golden proportion: the golden proportion of the width of the upper teeth displayed on a frontal view upon smiling is a recurrent 62% proportion – the width of the upper lateral incisor displayed should be 62% of the upper central incisor, the apparent width of the upper canine must be 62% of the upper lateral incisor and the first upper premolar apparent width should be 62% of the upper canine.

- ○ Black triangles: these are the gingival embrasures contour around the interproximal contacts in an aesthetically pleasing smile. Short interdental papillae fail to contour the interproximal contacts, so black triangles develop. Black triangles may occur as a result of periodontal disease and are commonly seen after correction of severely crowded or rotated teeth.
- ○ Buccal corridors: the smile width can be assessed by checking the degree of the first upper premolar exposure. The buccal corridor is the space formed between the inner buccal surfaces and the maxillary molars upon smiling. An aesthetically pleasing smile has reduced buccal corridors (Moore, 2005). The anteroposterior position of the maxilla and the inclination of the upper molars influence the width of the buccal corridor. Increased arch width results in reduced buccal corridor. Palatally inclined molars results in increased buccal corridor width.
- ○ Smile arc: There are three types of smile arcs:
  - Consonant: the border of the lower lip follows a curvature along the upper incisal edges. This is considered an ideal smile arc.
  - Flat: the superior boarder of the lower lip is parallel to the upper incisal edges.
  - Non-consonant: the top border of the lower lip forms a reverse curve with the upper incisal edges.
- Tongue: check for tongue thrust during speech or swallowing. Tongue thrust is protrusion of the tongue between the incisors due to musculature imbalance.

## Intraoral Examination

The purpose of this part of the examination is:

- to address chief compliant
- to determine clinical signs of malocclusion or dentoalveolar discrepancies
- to check periodontal health
- to assess the patient's oral health and hygiene status.

A systematic approach is needed to prevent omission. The intraoral examination commences with an assessment of the soft and hard tissue for any lesions, congenital abnormalities and evaluation of the occlusal relationships. Orthodontists assess four areas to make a diagnosis of the malocclusion:

1) Upper jaw
2) Upper dentoalveolar
3) Lower dentoalveolar
4) Lower jaw

The anteroposterior, vertical and transverse relationships of the alveolar bone, dentition and the underlying basal bone forms the final diagnosis.

## Soft Tissues

In a logical approach, all the soft tissues in the mouth must be assessed for any abnormalities. Using a good source of light, dental mirror and a probe, examine:

- the oral mucosa and vestibules
- the glands
- the fraenum
- the health status of the gingiva

- the gingival margins
- the soft and hard palate
- the tongue.

A periodontal chart is also recommended for patients presenting with signs of poor periodontal health. In cases of any form of periodontal disease, orthodontic treatment is contraindicated until the disease is under control, regardless of the age of the patient.

### Hard Tissues

Teeth must be charted carefully and all findings must be recorded thoroughly. The clinical examination must have a systematic routine to ensure that nothing is missed. It is recommended to begin the examination from one quadrant and move across to the next, assessing and recording:

- the presence of pathology
- detected caries
- erupted teeth
- enamel morphology
- missing teeth and reason for tooth loos
- previous dental treatment
- previous or current trauma.

It is extremely important to note the pattern of eruption to assess the dental age. Delayed eruptions, particularly asymmetrical delayed eruptions, may indicate an underlying problem such as a supernumerary teeth, ectopic eruption or impaction (see Chapter 6). The area must be palpated for permanent successors both palatally, lingually and labially. Radiographs are necessary if the permanent successor is not palpable. However, further data collection may be required in patients with a history of trauma, as the tooth may be dilacerated (bent roots), resulting in a delayed eruption.

### Occlusion

Occlusion is the relationship between the upper and lower jaws. Various terminologies are given to the occlusion depending on how the jaws meet. When the teeth meet during a function, such as speech or eating, the occlusion is termed 'dynamic occlusion'. The centric relation is critical during an intraoral examination. The centric relation is the most posterior position of the mandible. In centric relation, the mandibular condyle is in the most superior and posterior position in the glenoid fossa. The centric relation is considered the orthodontic problem. The centric occlusion refers to the habitual bite or bite of comfort. Centric occlusion is also known as intercuspation position, because of the maximum interdigitation as the cusps of both arches lock in completely.

### Dentoalveolar Compensations

When noting malocclusion and skeletal patterns, attention must be paid to dentoalveolar compensations. The dentoalveolar compensatory mechanism is when discrepancies are camouflaged or disguised due to dentoalveolar modifications; for example, protrusive upper anterior incisors camouflaging the severity of a skeletal class III malocclusion.

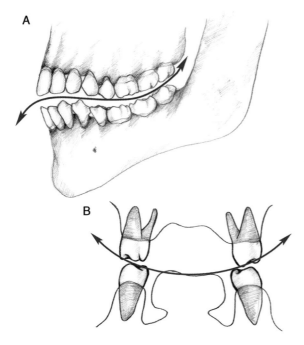

Figure 3.5  Types of occlusal curvature: A) Curve of Spee. B) Curve of Wilson.

**Midline Shift**
Check the path of mandibular closure to assess the midline when the patient bites into maximum interdigitation. Any displacement or deviation upon closure is best examined from behind, looking directly down from above the patient. The patient must therefore be in a supine position.

**Occlusal Curvature**
Another critical aspect to be noted is the curvature of the occlusion. An ideal occlusion contains a flat occlusal plane. The various types of occlusal curvature are:

- the curve of Spee: a curvature in the mandible caused by extrusion of the anterior teeth and intrusion of the molar teeth. It is typically seen in deep bites (Figure 3.5a).
- the curve of Wilson: a curvature in the occlusion resulting from inward tipping of the molars (Figure 3.5b).

**Occlusal Relationships**
The canine and molar occlusal relationships are best assessed using Angle's classification and the incisor relationships examined on the basis of the British standards incisor classification (Table 3.2). In an ideal occlusion, all lower teeth are about half a unit anterior to the upper teeth (Figure 3.6). This is because of the size differences between the upper and lower incisors; the lower anterior teeth are narrower than the upper anterior teeth.

***Class I Malocclusion***   Class I represents the ideal occlusion. Orthodontists aim to achieve class I molar, canine and incisor relationships when planning any treatment (Figure 3.7).

**Table 3.2** Assessment of canine and molar occlusal relationships: Angle's classification and the British standard classification of incisor relationships.

| Classification | Class I<br>Neutrocclusion | Class II<br>Distocclusion | Class III<br>Mesiocclusion |
|---|---|---|---|
| *Angle's Classification* | | | |
| Molar relationship | The mesiobuccal cusp of the upper first molar occludes on the mesiobuccal groove of the lower first molar. | The lower first molar is positioned distal to the upper first molar. | The lower first molar is positioned mesial to the upper first molar. |
| Canine relationship | Upper canine occludes on the mesial half of the lower first premolar and the distal half of the lower canine. | Upper canine occludes anteriorly to the lower first premolar. Thus, the distal surface of the lower canine lies posteriorly to the mesial surface of the upper canine by width of a premolar. If it is less than width of a premolar it is given the term 'tendency towards class II'. | The distal surface of the lower canine lies anteriorly to the mesial surface of the upper canine by width of a premolar. If it is less than width of a premolar it is given the term 'tendency towards class III'. |
| *British Standard Classification of Incisor Relationship* | | | |
| Relationship | The lower incisor edges occlude with or lie immediately below the cingulum of the upper central incisors. | The lower incisor edges lie posterior to the cingulum of the upper incisors. There are two subdivisions to this classification. The first division is protrusion of the incisors resulting in an overjet and the second division results in a deep bite as the upper central incisors are retroclined. | The lower incisors lie anterior to the upper central incisors. There is reduced or reverse overjet. |

However, a class I malocclusion can present with normal molar, canine or incisor relationship but discrepancies within the arches may be evident. The common problems are dental-related issues rather than skeletal abnormalities, with the exception of bimaxillary cases. The list below covers some of the most common findings in class I malocclusion that require significant attention during examination. These findings can be evident in combination with class II and class III malocclusions and are not confined to class I malocclusion.

- Crowding and spacing.: the lack of space results in crowding and occurs as the maxilla and/or the mandible fail to accommodate for any size discrepancies between the dental arches and the teeth. Extra spacing can be related to microdontia (teeth smaller than the normal size), tooth loss or hypodontia (congenitally missing teeth).
- Rotations: teeth that are rotated in the socket.
- Ankylosis: this is the term used to describe fusion of roots to the alveolar bone. Ankylosis is commonly seen in overretained deciduous teeth with missing permanent successors.

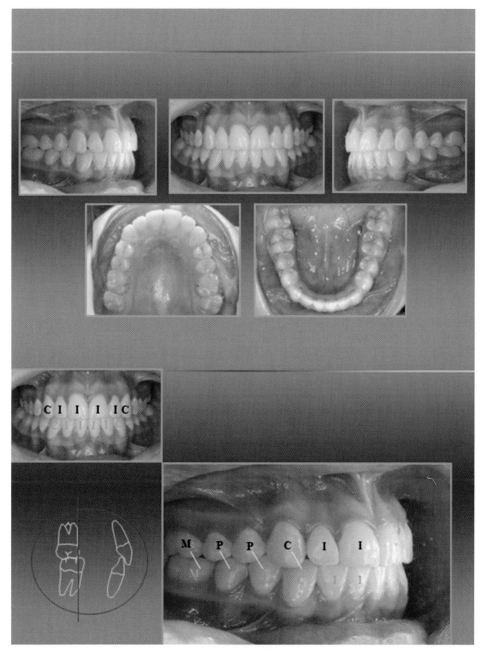

Figure 3.6 Normal occlusion. *Source*: Illustration by Professor Ali Darendeliler.

- Cross bite (Figure 3.8A): this is commonly seen in patients with a narrow maxilla. Cross bite occurs when maxillary teeth are positioned lingually in relation to the mandibular teeth. It can occur anteriorly or posteriorly and may involve one tooth or a group of teeth.

- Scissor bite (Figure 3.8B): the maxillary teeth rest completely outside or inside the mandibular teeth.
- Impacted teeth: blockage of an erupting tooth is called impaction. The most commonly impacted teeth are the third permanent molars and canines.
- Ectopic teeth (Figure 3.9): teeth erupting or located in an unusual position.

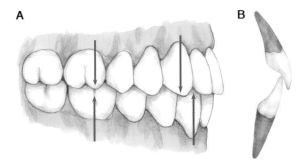

Figure 3.7 Class I: A) molar and canine relationship. B) Class I Incisor relationship. *Source*: Courtesy of professor Ali Darendeliler.

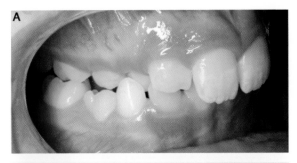

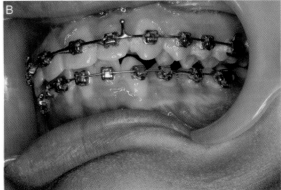

Figure 3.8 Class I malocclusions: A) Cross bite. B) Scissor bite.

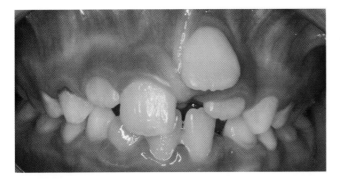

Figure 3.9 Ectopic central incisor.

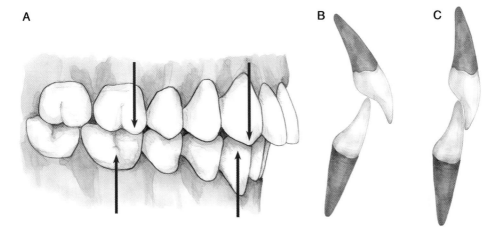

Figure 3.10 Class II: A) Molar and canine relationship. B) Incisor relationship, division 1. C) Incisor relationship, division 2.

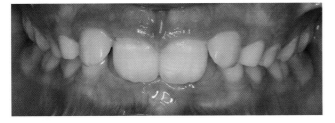

Figure 3.11 Class II division 2; retroclined upper central incisors with proclined lateral incisors.

*Class II Malocclusion*   Class II malocclusion is shown in Figure 3.10. Within class II, a division 1 malocclusion is an increased overjet with proclined upper central incisors (Figure 3.10B). A division 2 malocclusion is an increased overbite with retroclined upper central incisors (Figure 3.10C). The upper lateral incisors overlap the central incisors in some cases (Figure 3.11).

A                                                                                    B

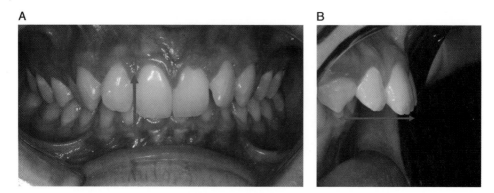

**Figure 3.12** A) 100% overbite. B) Overjet.

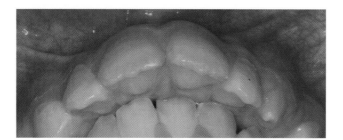

**Figure 3.13** Traumatic bite.

Patients with class II skeletal patterns tend to position the mandible forwards to reduce the degree of overjet and to disguise the underlying problem. This false bite is known as a Sunday bite. When assessing the profile and examining the occlusion, check that the mandible is not positioned too far forward.

Overjet is the horizontal discrepancy between the upper and lower incisors measured in millimetres (Figure 3.12B). In cases of severe overjet, the lower incisal edges will bite in the soft tissue of the maxillary anterior region (Figure 3.13). This traumatic bite will lead to gingival ulceration and recession if left untreated. Overbite is the vertical discrepancy between the upper and lower incisors measured in percentages (Figure 3.12A).

***Class III Malocclusion***   Class III malocclusion is shown in Figure 3.14. In some cases, the patients can achieve an edge-to-edge bite but, once at rest, the lower incisors can slip forwards, resulting in a reverse jet. This bite is called pseudo class III, as the patient does not have a true class III malocclusion, meaning the centric relation is edge to edge as the mandible is in its most posterior position (Figure 3.15). However, the centric occlusion as the habitual bite of the patient slips into a class III, as the mandible protrudes forward to achieve maximum interdigitation.

### Primary Dentition
The permanent and primary dentition share the same classification for incisor and canine relationships but the molar classification is assessed on the terminal plane, based

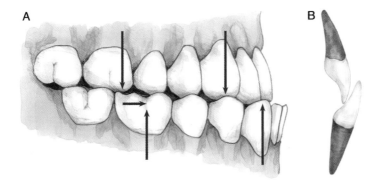

Figure 3.14 Class III malocclusion: A) Molar and canine relationship. B) Incisor relationship.

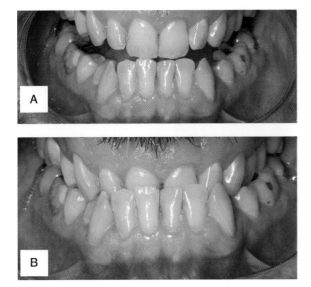

Figure 3.15 Pseudo class III: A) Centric relation: edge to edge bite. B) Centric occlusion.

on the relative position of the upper and lower second primary molars in a vertical plane (Figure 3.16).

1) Flush terminal plane: the distal of the primary mandibular second molar lies in line with the distal of the primary upper second molar (same vertical plane). This can lead to a class I or a class II molar relationship in the permanent dentition.
2) Distal step: the distal of the primary mandibular second molar lies distal to the primary upper second molar. A class II molar relationship is predictable in the permanent dentition.
3) Mesial step: the distal surface of the primary mandibular second molar lies mesial to the primary upper second molar. Studies reveal that this type of occlusion typically results in a class I molar relationship in the permanent dentition. However, if the mesial step is greater than 2 mm, a class III molar relationship is inevitable.

**1**   **2**   **3**

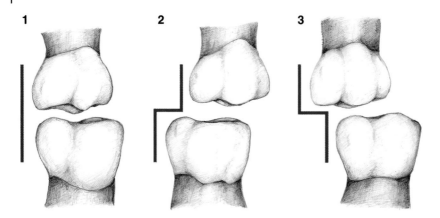

Figure 3.16 Terminal planes: 1) Flush terminal plane. 2) Distal step. 3) Mesial step.

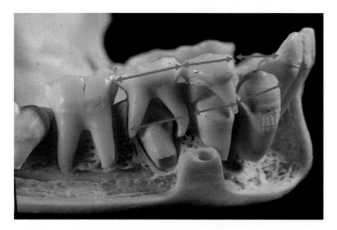

Figure 3.17 Leeway spaces: the differences in the mesiodistal width between the primary teeth and their permanent successors. *Source*: Courtesy of Professor Ali Darendeliler.

### Leeway and Primate Spaces

The difference in the mesiodistal width between the primary teeth and their permanent successors is known as the leeway spaces (Figures 3.17). The total width of primary canines, first and second primary molars is greater than the total width of permanent canines, first and second premolars. In the upper arch, there is an average of 1–1.5 mm excess space per quadrant and in the lower arch there is an average of 2–2.5 mm of excessive space per quadrant. These space discrepancies can be used in relieving minor crowding to a degree in the permanent dentition.

Spacing in the primary dentition is common and expected. Space is commonly detected mesial to the maxillary canine and distal to the mandibular canines. These spaces are known as primate spaces (Figure 3.18). Generally, crowding is expected in the permanent dentition if spacing is not evident once the primary dentition is established.

A
B

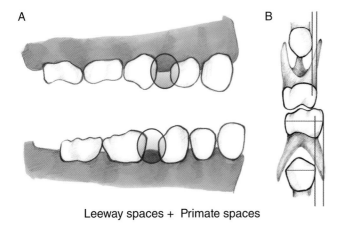

Leeway spaces + Primate spaces

Figure 3.18  A) Primate spaces. B) Example of leeway spaces; the mesiodistal width of the deciduous molars is larger than the width of the permanent premolars.

**Mixed dentition**

The term 'mixed dentition' is given to a dentition where the both permanent and primary teeth are present. Early detection of malocclusion aids in prevention of complex orthodontic treatment in the later stages of growth and development. The eruption of permanent teeth should be monitored to detect any signs of abnormalities in the pattern of eruption during the early mixed dentition stage.

The early mixed dentition stage begins with eruption of the first permanent molars and lower incisors around the age of six years. Several factors influence this stage of development and affect the direction of eruption of the lower incisors:

- rotation of growth
- soft tissue
- habits.

The late mixed dentition stage commences with the eruption of the lower canines and the upper and lower first premolars at the age of eleven years.

Between the ages of 7 and 12 years, children may undergo a phase known as the 'ugly duckling' stage (also known as the Broadbent phenomenon, after B. H. Broadbent, who first described it in 1937). A median diastema (space in the midline) occurs, with protrusion and lateral spacing of the upper incisors preceding the eruption of the maxillary canines. As the upper canines erupt, the incisors mesialise and the closure of the diastema becomes evident. This can be monitored and active orthodontic treatment is generally not indicated unless it is accompanied by an underlying skeletal discrepancy.

From the ages of 8–10 years of age, the presence of canine successors should be palpable in the sulcus of both upper and lower arches. Radiographs are indicated if delayed eruption is noticed or the permanent successors are not palpable. Negligence in monitoring the pattern of eruption leads to irrevocable consequences. In Figure 3.19, an ectopic canine was not detected at an early stage. The ectopic upper left canine

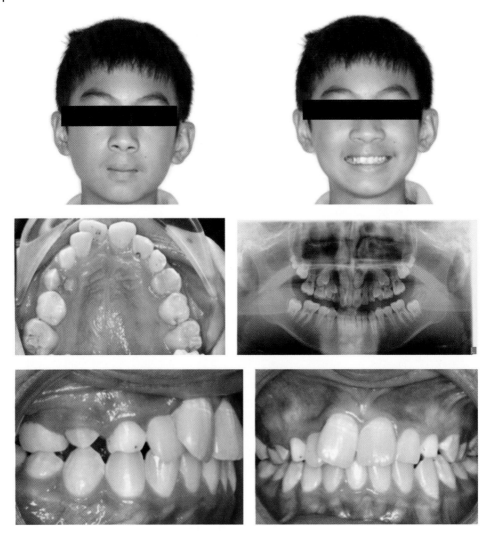

**Figure 3.19** Ectopic canine not detected at an early stage; initial records. *Source*: Case by Dr Jim Bokas.

resorbed the root of the upper left central incisor (Figure 3.20). Saving the incisor became impossible for the orthodontist as more than one-third of the root was resorbed and a significant degree of mobility was evident clinically. Extraction of the upper left central incisor and the overretained deciduous canines was indicated to create space for the eruption of the canine into the central incisor space. This technique is known as transposition.

Once the canine was erupted and aligned into position, cosmetic restorations were used to alter the shape of the canine to resemble the central incisor and final alignment and space closure was achieved (Figure 3.21–3.23).

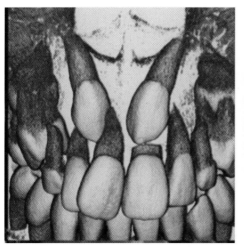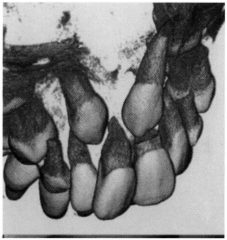

Figure 3.20 Three-dimensional scan of the ectopic canine reveals the damage that it has caused to the upper left central incisor. *Source*: Courtesy of Dr. Jim Bokas.

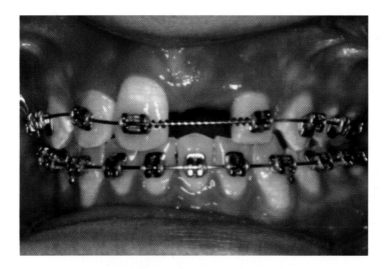

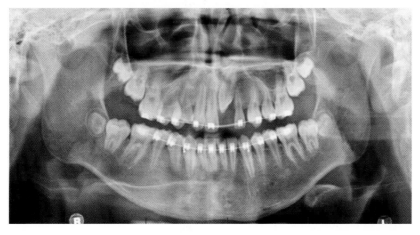

Figure 3.21 Space was created using fixed appliances to allow eruption of the upper left canine in the central incisor position. This is termed transposition. *Source*: Courtesy of Dr. Jim Bokas.

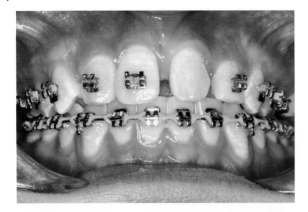

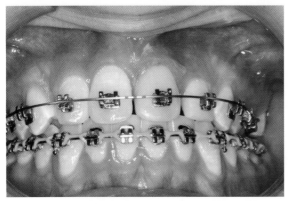

Figure 3.22 Composite resin restoration of the canine was indicated to resemble the central incisor.

## Records

Dental photographs and models of teeth are valuable diagnostic tools in orthodontics. In this section, the essentials for quality photographs and dental impressions are discussed.

### Photographs

Dental photographs are essential medico-legal documents and have other major benefits such as marketing, communication among practitioners and patient education. Thus, the quality of the photographs must be of a high standard. These photographs not only provide valuable baseline data in practices but also create a visual record of the orthodontic problem of the patient and aid in the acceptance of treatment.

To document accurate pre- and post-treatment photographs of a high standard, the clinician must learn to control and standardise the variables. These variables include technique, patient positioning and selection of camera, lens and flash. Photographs within the oral cavity are termed intraoral photographs and photographs of the head and neck are extra oral photographs (Figure 3.24).

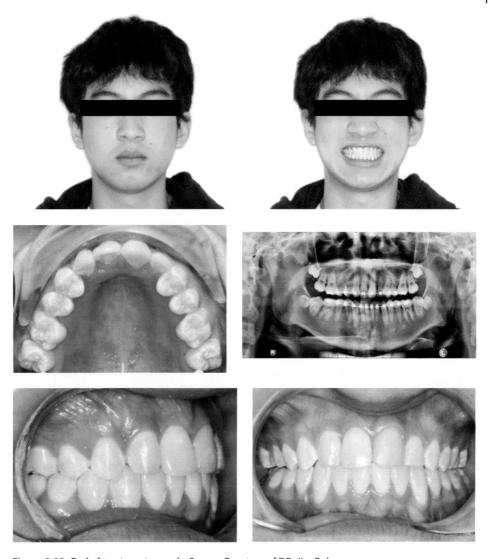

Figure 3.23 End of treatment records. *Source*: Courtesy of DR. Jim Bokas.

**The Camera**

Camera selection plays an important role in achieving a high standard of photographic record. A digital single lens reflex (DSLR) camera is an ideal choice. Other cameras may require extra equipment to adapt them to be appropriate for dental photography. Lens and flash selection also require specific attention. Macro lenses allow close distance photographs taken without affecting the quality of the image.

The following must be considered for capturing clinical photographs:

- Focus: all images must clearly show the required detail. If an image is blurred, it is out of focus. By turning the focus ring, the image will sharpen.

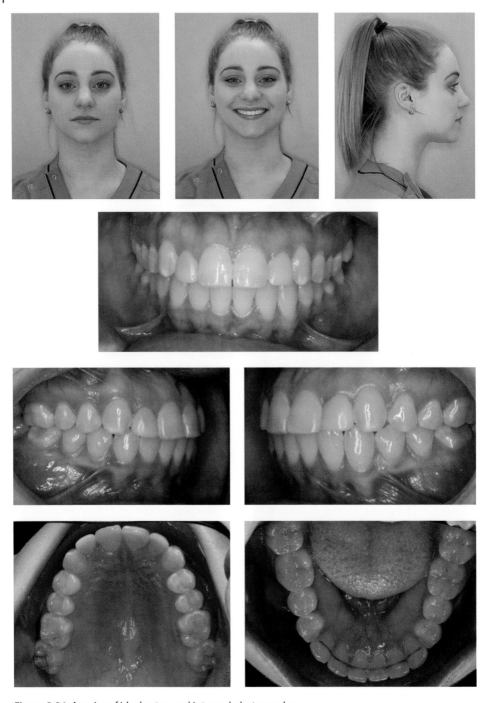

Figure 3.24  A series of ideal extra- and intraoral photographs.

- Exposure: the images must have sufficient light. The exposure is determined by luminesce of the area, shutter speed, ISO setting and lens aperture. Shutter speed is the exposure duration, controlling the amount of time the sensor is exposed to light. ISO settings control the sensitivity of the sensor to the light. Sensitivity is reduced with lower ISO. If sensitivity is high due to an increased ISO, images will have grains or 'noise' added to it. Generally, ISO is increased in low luminesce areas. Aperture controls the amount of light passing through the lens and it is known as the f-stop value. The depth of field is dependent on the aperture. The lower the aperture, the shallower the depth of field as more light will pass through the lens.
- Framing: capturing the subject only. Capturing the top of the head up to the shoulders is sufficient for the extra oral photographs. Intraoral photographs must clearly show all the hard and soft tissues.

### Settings

The DSLR camera offers several settings. All exposure settings will be preselected if the camera is set to automatic. In the manual mode, all three variables of shutter speed, ISO setting and aperture must be set as required for the image being captured. The author recommends the following for quality photographs on a manual setting:

- ISO – 1/60 seconds
- extraoral – lower aperture (f); e.g., 5.6
- intraoral – higher aperture (f); e.g., 22.

The setting can greatly vary, depending on the type of camera used. Every specialist will have their own preferred setting for capturing clinical photographs.

### Technique

***Extraoral Photographs*** Extraoral photographs should be obtained against a plain background with the camera held at 90 degrees (Figure 3.25A). The posture of the patient plays a major role in the accuracy of the photographs. The patient should be in a relaxed neutral position, with the chin parallel to the floor and the eyes focused on the lens. The top of the head, forehead, ears and base of the neck must clearly be visible, excluding the shoulders. Hair should be tied back and any items covering the face and neck must be

A                                  B

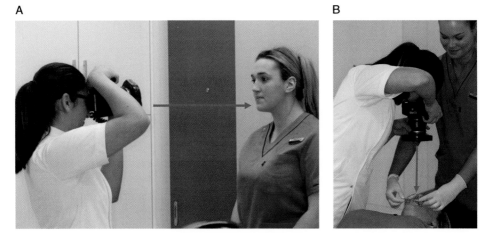

Figure 3.25 Camera position for: A) Extraoral photographs. B) Intraoral photographs.

removed, such as glasses, scarf or hat. One photograph should be taken with the patient in a resting position with relaxed facial muscles and a second with the patient smiling and biting in maximum interdigitation. Some orthodontists may also request a close-up of the smile for further assessment of the smile. Another photograph is needed of the lateral profile of the patient in a relaxed position, for assessment of the skeletal pattern and facial profile. To assess the social smile framework, the patient can be asked to slightly turn from the profile position to capture a 45-degree profile, also known as three-quarter profile.

*Intraoral Photographs*   The patient must be seated comfortably in a supine or semi-supine position for intraoral photographs (Figure 3.25B). It is crucial that the camera is positioned directly above the patient. Cheek retractors are used to retract the cheeks and lips, allowing a better field of view of the occlusion. Three photographs are taken:

- centre occlusion
- left occlusion
- right occlusion.

It is extremely important that the first molars are visible in photographs showing molar relationships. Lip retractors move the upper or lower lip away from the teeth as intraoral mirrors are placed posterior to the last erupted molar (Figures 3.26 and 3.27). A photograph of the reflection provides upper and lower occlusal views. To prevent the dental mirrors from becoming foggy, ask the patient to breathe through their nose and the mirror must be kept in warm water before insertion into the mouth. To avoid trauma and burn to the intraoral tissues, ensure that the mirror is cooled down before inserting it into the mouth. It is also important to notify the patient of all the steps involved for better patient management. Guiding the patient also enhances patient cooperation.

In extraoral photographs, common errors include:

- Poor patient posture – the patient should not slouch.
- Incorrect head and neck position – the head must be in a neutral position. Care must be given the head and neck are not positioned too far back, too low or tilted.
- The chin and forehead must be relaxed in all the photographs.
- Hair covering the forehead and face – hair must be tied back to make the face, ears and neck visible.
- Not capturing the base of the neck.
- Out of focus images.
- Incorrect framing.

In intraoral photographs, common errors include:

- Not capturing all the critical intraoral structures.
- Poor cheek and lip retraction results in coverage of the roots and the mucogingival areas by the lips.
- Incorrectly sized intraoral mirrors and retractors can be uncomfortable for the patient and can cause insufficient retraction.
- Incorrect camera angulation – the image will not be accurate.
- Incorrect patient positioning – the angulation of the image is affected if the patient's head is positioned too far upwards or downwards.
- Out of focus images.

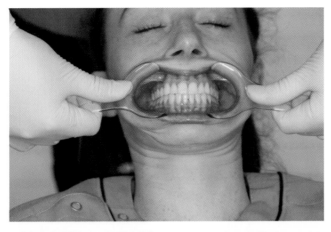

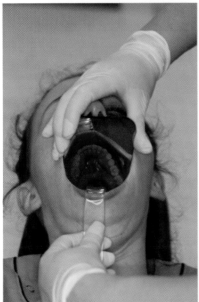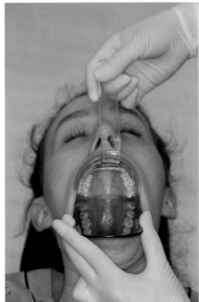

**Figure 3.26** Intraoral photography accessories: cheek retractors (top), lip retractor and occlusal mirror (bottom).

### Impressions and Digital Scanners

Dental impressions provide an imprint of the teeth, gingiva and surrounding tissues. A positive model is created once the alginate impressions are poured with plaster to achieve a replica of the oral tissues. Cast models are used as a diagnostic tool and fabrication of appliances. Therefore, the quality and accuracy of the impressions are critical (Figure 3.28).

### Impression Trays

Choosing a correct impression tray size is the first step to a great impression. The trays are either plastic or metal (autoclavable). Perforations in the trays enhance the adhesion

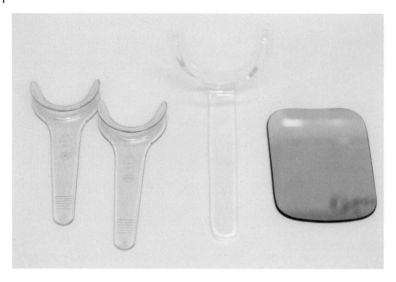

Figure 3.27 Intraoral photography accessories.

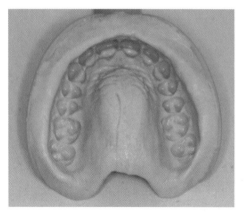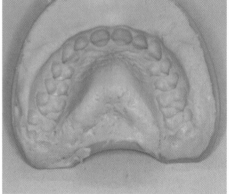

Figure 3.28 Ideal impression on the left side, showing sufficient detail of hard and soft tissue coverage. On the right side, there is dragging of the posterior region, sufficient details are not captured and the impression material mix was of a poor quality as it was set prior to insertion so the teeth are not fully captured.

of the alginate to the tray. To increase the retention and prevent separation of the material from the tray, adhesives are brushed on the inner surfaces of the tray before loading the alginate material.

### Impression Materials

The impression materials are classified as non-elastic and elastic. Non-elastic materials are plaster and wax. Elastic materials are further categorised as synthetic elastomers and hydrocolloids.

*Elastomers*   Polysulfide, silicone and polyether are three different types of synthetic elastomers. These are manufactured in three different viscosities of light body with low viscosity, medium/regular body and heavy body, which has the highest viscosity. Silicone is classified based on its polymerisation method. Type I is condensation curing and type II is addition curing. Putty materials are a type of silicone that are extremely viscous and consist of a much higher filler content than the heavy-body silicone. Putty was invented to reduce the shrinkage effect upon polymerisation of the material due to its higher filler content. Typically, putty is used in combination with a low-viscosity silicone in a putty wash technique (discussed in the technique section). Polysulfide and condensation-cured silicone have comparable physical properties, although polyether and addition-cured silicone similarly present better dimensional stabilities. The maximum storage time for synthetic elastomers is around 48 hours.

*Hydrocolloids*   There are two types of hydrocolloid dental impressions: agar and alginate. Agar can repeatedly reverse between high-viscosity gel and low-viscosity solution with temperature changes. Agar is not commonly used in the dental setting, as it requires complex set-up and armamentarium. Alginate is irreversible, as it will not convert back into solution after gelation. Alginate is non-toxic, non-irritant and inexpensive. It is therefore widely used in dental practice. Hydrocolloids are hydrophilic with insufficient tear resistance and poor dimensional stability (Walls, 2002). Over the years, manufacturers have produced dust-free alginate materials with improved formulas that provide better physical properties to enhance the accuracy and stability of the material.

### Alginate Setting Reaction
Alginate is in a form of a powder composed of sodium alginate, calcium sulphate, trisodium phosphate, diatomaceous earth, zinc oxide and potassium titanium fluoride (Nandini, 2008). Once mixed with water, a chemical reaction between the soluble alginate and the calcium sulphate occurs, resulting in the production of a gel gel-like insoluble calcium alginate. The setting rate of this reaction can be controlled by water temperature. The higher the temperature of the water, the faster the material sets. Trisodium phosphate is incorporated into the material to slow down the chemical reaction and increase working time. Some alginate materials are manufactured with a colour change setting indicator, meaning it will change colour upon setting.

### Mixing and Loading Alginate
The powder to water ratio can vary, depending on the manufacturer's guidelines.

Using a flat spatula, the content must be mixed rapidly. To prevent air bubbles becoming trapped in the material, smear the mix against the mixing bowl. The aim is to achieve an alginate mix that is smooth and viscose. The alginate mix becomes runny with excessive water or dry and hard to mix with insufficient water. The impression trays must be loaded with adequate material. The excess is to be removed from the edges of the tray and over the surface.

### Technique
The initial step is to decide on the correct tray size for the dental arch, regardless of the type of material used. In the upper arch, the trays must cover the hard palate, maxillary

tuberosity and the vestibular areas. In the lower arch, the tray must cover the mandibular retromolar area, lingual fraenum, tongue space, vestibular area and the mylohyoid ridge. Anteriorly, there must be about a 5 mm space for the material to fill in the vestibular areas. The edges of the trays are usually covered with peripheral wax for better patient comfort and act as an extension to the tray. Prior to loading the material on to the impression trays, an adhesive is brushed over the inner surfaces to prevent separation of the material upon removal.

***Alginate impressions***   Its best to take the lower impression first, as the upper impression induces a gagging reflex in many patients. There are two ways in which impressions can be taken:

1) Keeping the patient in a supine position.
2) Keeping the patient sitting upright.

Both positions can have advantages for the patient and the practitioner. Keeping the patient in a supine position provides a better field of vision for the practitioner and thus better placement of the impression tray, particularly in the upper. Sitting upright position can be more comfortable for the patient, particularly those with a strong gag reflex.

For a better field of vision and positioning of the trays, it is best to stand behind the patient for the upper impression (Figure 3.29A) and in front of the patient to take the

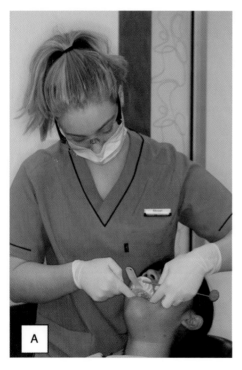
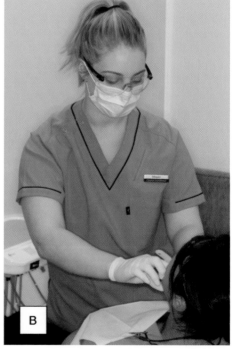

**Figure 3.29** Taking an impression: A) Standing behind the patient for the upper. B) Standing in front of the patient for the lower impression for a better field of vision.

lower impression (Figure 3.29B). Use a dental mirror to retract the cheek and lip. Always insert the trays in sideways first to avoid overstretching the labial commissures. Always seat the impression on the posterior teeth first and slowly seat the anterior, with no movement once the tray is positioned. Any movement after the tray is seated will cause distortion to the impression.

Ensure that teeth are not desiccated, as the radicals from the chemical reactions in the material tend to bond with enamel hydroxyapatite. Thus, removal of the impression will be difficult or may result in tear of the material. If the impressions are required on patients with braces, it is important to cover it with dental wax to prevent tear of the alginate upon removal.

Impressions are not pleasant for patients and cause a gagging reflex, particularly if the impression reaches the soft palate. It may also be psychologically induced, particularly in anxious patients. The best strategy for managing patients during this procedure is to help patients control their breathing pattern. Slow deep breaths through the nose can aid in managing anxious patients and are an expedient distraction.

### Putty wash
The putty-wash technique can be obtained in three methods:

1) Laminate technique – this is a one-stage impression technique, as both putty and wash are recorded instantaneously. This technique is also termed twin mix.
2) Two-stage unspaced – putty is loaded in the dental tray and seated on the mouth. A thin layer of wash is lined over the set putty and reinserted in the mouth.
3) Two-staged spaced – once the putty is recorded and set, a space is created for the wash with either polyethylene spacer over the teeth before the putty impression is taken or making indentations in the putty to create channels for outflow of the wash.

### Bite Registration
Bite registration is essential, particularly for study models. Diagnosis becomes difficult for orthodontists if an incorrect bite is registered. Fabrication of some appliances also requires bite registration; thus, incorrect technique will lead to poor fit of the appliance. A non-elastic impression material such as wax is typically used for bite registration. The wax is trimmed into small rectangles and softened in warm water before insertion in the mouth. Polyvinyl siloxane (PVS) can also be used to obtain bite registration. Monitor the patient closely to ensure that the correct bite is captured. It is best to position the wax posteriorly on the occlusal table for better vision of the incisal relationships. If the wax covers too much of the anterior region, it will be difficult to check for the correct occlusion. Capturing the molars and canines is usually sufficient for a quality bite registration.

### Disinfection and Storage
All dental impressions must be disinfected prior to any laboratory preparations to prevent cross contamination without causing distortions to the impressions. Once removed from the mouth, impressions must thoroughly be rinsed under cold running water to remove saliva, debris and blood. Studies suggest that all impressions should be immersed in 1% sodium hypochlorite for a minimum of ten minutes.

Inappropriate storage can cause distortion to the material, so it is recommended that the impressions are poured with plaster immediately or stored in cool temperatures in

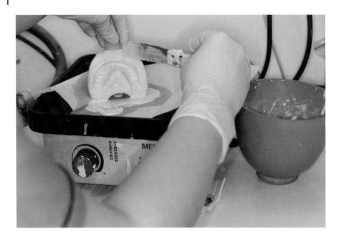

Figure 3.30  Pouring impressions with plaster of Paris.

damp tissues to prevent dehydration of the material. The impression dries out and shrinks if left in open air for a prolonged period of time. Evaporation of moisture from the impression is termed syneresis. If the material is left in excessive water, it swells and expands, which is known as imbibition.

### Cast Models

The impressions are poured with a non-elastic impression material such as plaster of Paris to achieve a positive of the impressions (Figure 3.30). These casts are used as records, study models or fabrication of appliances. The plaster is mixed with water similarly to alginate. The water and plaster ratio can vary depending on the manufacturing guidelines. To avoid air bubbles in the final cast models, a dental plaster vibrator machine is used in laboratories. The impression trays are placed over the machine and plaster is poured from one end of the impression until all teeth are covered with the material. The base of the material should have a thicker consistency, so a higher powder to water ratio is needed to create the base. These are left to set over time and trimmed once hardened (Figure 3.31).

### Common Errors

To guarantee high standards, practitioners must examine each impression thoroughly prior to disinfection and storage. Some of the common errors include:

- separation of the material from the tray
- voids or drags
- air bubbles in the impression
- syneresis or imbibition due to improper storage
- removal of impression from the mouth prior to setting results in an inaccurate impression
- air bubbles in cast models due to incorrect technique
- breakage of models during separation of the impression trays from the models (the models are prone to breakage if the material is still soft if it is not set).

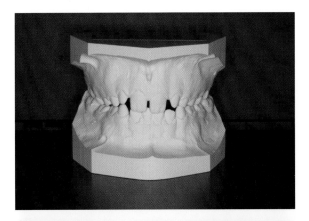

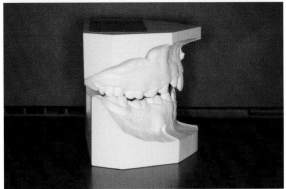

**Figure 3.31** Trimmed plaster models.

### Digital Scanners

Over the years, there has been a paradigm shift in taking dental impressions and cast models in dentistry. In many practices, digital scanners have replaced dental impressions (Figures 3.32 and 3.33). The digital scans are sent to digital laboratories to produce three-dimensional models of the digital data. This innovative technology has several advantages in comparison with conventional impressions and plaster models. Advantages are:

- greater accuracy
- better patient comfort
- digital storage of models
- eliminates the risk of cross contamination.

There are four types of imaging technology (Kravitz, 2014):

1) Triangulation uses laser light to measure angles and distances used in CEREC (Chairside Economical Restoration of aEsthetic Ceramics, or CEramic REConstruction).
2) Parallel confocal imaging uses laser and optical scanning to capture intraoral structures.
3) Accordion fringe interferometry.
4) Three-dimensional in-motion video.

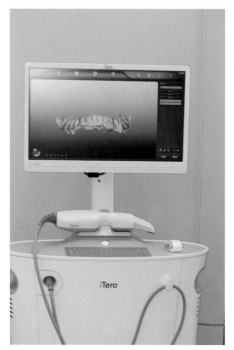
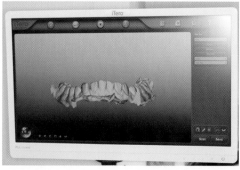
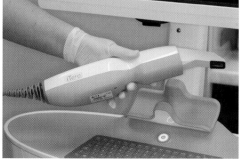

Figure 3.32 Digital scanner; the iTero machine uses a powder-free technology for accurate scanning; a gentle stream of air disperses from the wand.

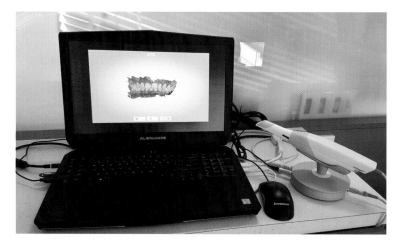

Figure 3.33 The TRIOS POD is another example of a digital scanner. This innovative technology is a much smaller scanner with dramatically reduced chair time and provides more patient comfort. This scanner can easily be connected to multiple laptops or computers and the pod solution allows the scanner to easily be relocated and shared among various treatment rooms.

Some digital scanners may require the application of a layer of powder to eliminate any inconsistencies caused by tooth and restorative surfaces dispersing light at an impulsive angle. The powder is commonly composed of titanium oxide or zirconium oxide with amorphous silica and aluminium hydroxide. This technique is termed dusting or accent frosting.

### Analysis of Study Models

The diagnostic models retrieved either from dental impressions or digital scanners are analysed for occlusal symmetry and space. The symmetry of each dental arch is assessed carefully by the orthodontist. An assessment of space is made during this part of the examination. Crowding is classified as mild, moderate or severe. The categories are:

- mild: 1–2 mm of crowding per quadrant
- moderate: up to 4 mm of crowding per quadrant
- severe: more than 4 mm of crowding per quadrant.

Space analysis allows a better comparison of the degree of space available in the dental arches with the space necessary for alignment of the dentition. The space available is calculated by a linear measurement of all four segments. The total sum of the mesiodistal width of every tooth in the arch is needed, including an estimation of the size of permanent teeth that have not yet erupted. There is a space deficiency in the arch if the total sum of the space required is higher than the space available in the arch.

### Radiographs

One of the most valuable diagnostic tools in orthodontics are radiographs. The two most important radiographs indicated for an accurate orthodontic diagnosis are orthopantomogram and lateral cephalometric radiograph.

### Orthopantomogram

The orthopantomogram, also known as a dental panoramic tomogram, is a critical diagnostic tool, as it shows upper and lower arches with surrounding structures (Figure 3.34). This type of extraoral radiograph is commonly taken prior to treatment to aid in accurate diagnosis and at the end of treatment to ensure that the crown and root positioning are ideal. This radiograph must be examined in a systematic approach, working from one side to the other assessing:

- the position and size of the permanent and primary teeth
- tooth development (dental age)
- missing (hypodontia) and extra (hyperdontia) teeth
- alveolar bone density and height
- root inclinations
- impacted or ectopic teeth
- presence of pathology.

### Cephalometric Radiographs

The cephalostat is an x-ray machine invented after the First World War by B. Holly Broadbent to take cephalometric radiographs (Mitchell, 2001). This type of radiograph

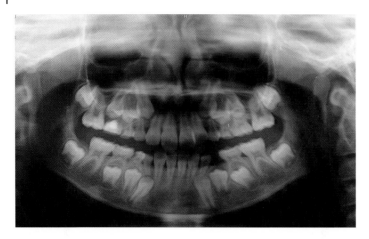

**Figure 3.34** Example of an orthopantomogram.

allows an assessment of the growth, balance and harmony of the dentofacial structures in various planes. Indications of lateral cephalometric radiographs and the different analyses are discussed briefly in this section. The objective of this section is to create a better understanding of the anatomical landmarks on lateral cephalometric radiographs and how it can aid an orthodontic diagnosis. However, as mentioned previously orthodontic diagnosis is solely the scope of an orthodontist.

This type of radiograph is not indicated for every orthodontic patient; however, it provides a valuable baseline record, particularly in patients with severe overjet. Lateral cephalometric radiographs at various stages of treatment allow a better assessment of the progress of treatment over time. It is important to examine airway patency, root length and any pathology on the radiograph prior to analysis of the skeletal discrepancies. Anatomical points and planes are used in the analysis (Figures 3.35, 3.36, 3.37 and Table 3.3). The relationship between the anatomical landmarks and points aid a radiographic diagnosis of any discrepancies.

The study of skeletal discrepancies and malocclusion on cephalometric radiographs dates back to 1934. Several analyses have been developed that assess the correlation of dental and skeletal structures using various methods. To provide a better understanding of the underlying dental and skeletal discrepancies and to measure the growing craniofacial structures, the analytical methods are categorised as angular or linear. The distance between the anatomical points is measured in millimetres and the angles formed between numerous points and planes are measured in degrees. The lateral cephalometric analysis can be manually hand traced, measured and calculated or digitised with software designed for this type of analysis.

Hand tracing involves tracing the outline of the soft tissue, anatomical landmarks and points over an acetate sheet secured to the x-ray. A light viewing box is necessary for accurate tracing. Once the points and planes are marked, the necessary angles and distances are measured according to the particular type of analysis used and a diagnosis is made. There are several computer programs designed to make cephalometric analysis easier and less time consuming. Once the landmarks are identified, the program will automatically identify the linear and angular measurements.

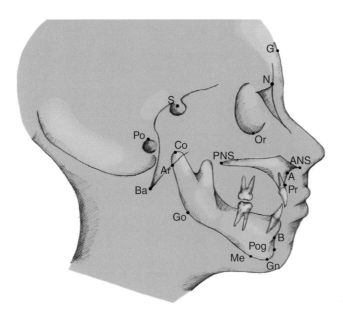

**Figure 3.35** Some commonly known anatomical landmarks and points; the same anatomical points are not used for all analyses. A, A-point (subspinale); ANS, anterior nasal spine; Ar, articular; B, B-point (supramentale); Ba, basion; Co, condylion; G, glabella; Gn, gnathion; Go, gonion; Me, menton; N, nasion; Or, orbitale; PNS, posterior nasal spine; Po, porion; Pog, pogonion; Pr, prosthion.

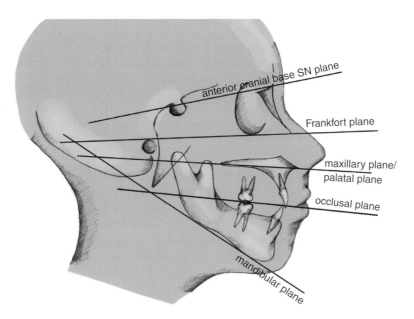

**Figure 3.36** Commonly used horizontal planes:

Anterior cranial base SN plane – a line from sella to nasion;
Frankfort plane – a line from orbitale to porion;
Maxillary or palatal plane – a line from the anterior nasal spine to the posterior nasal spine;
Occlusal plane – a line dividing the posterior occlusion;
Mandibular plane – a line from gonion to menton.

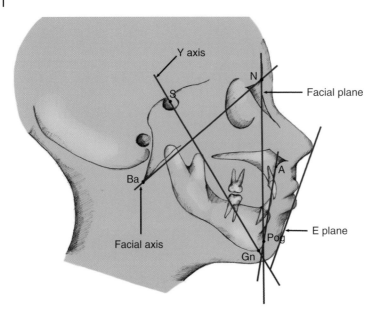

**Figure 3.37** Commonly used vertical planes:

> A–Pog line – a line from point A to pogonion;
> Facial plane – a line from nasion to pogonion;
> Facial axis – the x–y axis from the basion–nasion plane to the gnathion;
> Y-axis – a line from sella to gnathion; the angle formed between the y-axis and the Frankfort plane is an indication of facial growth tendency;
> E-plane – the aesthetic plane is a soft tissue plane from the base of the nose to the base of the chin.

Cephalometric analysis also creates a better understanding of which jaw presents with a discrepancy, as it may be difficult to accurately identify this clinically (Figure 3.38). The treatment will vary depending on which jaw is diagnosed with a skeletal malposition.

Patients with a high vertical skeletal angle are known as dolichocephalic, those with medium vertical skeletal angle are termed mesocephalic and those presenting with a low vertical skeletal angle are called brachycephalic (Alexander, 2008).

### Analyses

There are numerous cephalometric analyses developed to aid an orthodontic diagnosis. Each analysis has its advantages and disadvantages. A radiographic diagnosis is made by comparing the results of the traced lateral cephalometric radiographs to the chosen analyses. However, in contemporary orthodontics software programs are employed to achieve a radiographic diagnosis. Some of the common analyses include Steiner, Downs, Tweed, and McNamara; however, discussion of these analyses is beyond the scope of this textbook.

Table 3.3 Anatomical points and locations.

| Points | Symbol | Location |
| --- | --- | --- |
| A-point (subspinale) | A | The deepest part of the concavity between the anterior nasal spine and prosthions on the anterior portion of the maxilla. This point is located on the maxillary alveolar bone; thus, it varies over time with growth and bone remodelling due to tooth movement. |
| Anterior nasal spine | ANS | The most anterior portion of the nasal spine (bony process of the maxilla). |
| Articular | Ar | Junction between the posterior portion of the mandible and the basal part of the occipital bone. |
| B-point (supramentale) | B | The deepest part of the concavity between the alveolar crest of lower incisors and pogonion. |
| Basion | Ba | Anterior inferior portion of the foramen magnum. |
| Condylion | Co | The most superior point on the posterior part of the mandibular condyle. |
| Glabella | G | The most anterior portion of the prominence of the forehead. |
| Gnathion | Gn | The most posterior inferior portion of the symphysis (chin) – the midpoint of gonion and menton. |
| Gonion | Go | The lowest point on the angle of the mandible. |
| Menton | Me | The most inferior portion of the mandibular symphysis. |
| Nasion | N | The deepest point on the concavity at the junction of the frontal bone and the nasal bone. |
| Orbitale | Or | The lowest point on the anterior margin of the orbit. |
| Pogonion | Pog | The most anterior portion of the mandibular symphysis. |
| Porion | Po | The highest point of the external auditory meatus. |
| Posterior nasal spine | PNS | The most posterior portion of the nasal spine (bony process of maxilla). |
| Prosthion | Pr | The most anterior part of the maxillary alveolar process in the midline. |
| Sella | S | The centre of the Sella turcica, which is a depression in the sphenoid bone. |

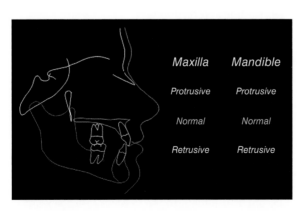

Figure 3.38 Sagittal jaw (skeletal) discrepancies. Radiographic diagnosis will confirm whether the jaws are in a normal position, retrusive or protrusive. A diagnosis is required for each jaw. *Source*: Courtesy of Professor Ali Darendeliler.

***Anteroposterior Radiographic Diagnosis*** Anteroposterior radiographic assessments are valuable diagnostic tools to identify transverse discrepancies in the maxilla and the mandible. Some common anteroposterior radiographic diagnoses based upon various radiographic analyses include:

- Sella–nasion–A point angle (SNA): 82 degrees – A protrusive maxilla is presented with a higher angle. A retrusive maxilla is presented with lower angle.
- Sella–nasion–B point angle (SNB): 80 degrees – A protrusive mandible is presented with a higher number. A retrusive mandible is presented with a lower number.
- A point–nasion–B point angle (ANB): 2 degrees. This angle is measured by calculating the difference between the SNA and the SNB. It is an indication of the anteroposterior discrepancy of the upper and lower arches. An ANB of 2–4 denotes class I, more than 4 is class II and less than 2 is class III.

***Wits analysis*** This appraisal was developed for cases where the ANB is unreliable and the clinical findings differ from the cephalometric reading. The lack of harmony in the anteroposterior relationship can be due to:

- the rotational effect of the jaws
- a reduction in ANB due to age
- the degree of mandibular protrusion
- a change of Sella–nasion angle to the occlusal plane
- alteration of the position of the nasion as a result of growth.

This analysis involves measuring the relative position of the mandible and the maxilla on a sagittal plane without comparison to other cranial landmarks. Two perpendicular lines join the occlusal plane from the A-point and B-point, labelled AO and BO, respectively. The occlusal plane is a line drawn along the cusp tips of the molars and premolars. According to Wits, the average jaw relationship is 1 mm in males and 0 mm in females. In skeletal class II, BO is located posterior to AO. In skeletal class III, BO is located anterior to AO. This type of analysis was developed as an extra diagnostic tool to enhance the accuracy of the anteroposterior relationships of the jaws and not as a single diagnostic criterion.

***Ballard Conversion*** The Ballard conversion is another alternative approach introduced where the clinical and cephalometric findings were different. Incisors are used as indicators to determine the anteroposterior relations of the maxilla and the mandible.

***The Bolton Analysis*** The Bolton tooth size analysis was developed by Wayne A. Bolton to examine any discrepancies in sizes of the maxillary and mandibular teeth. There are two elements to this analysis:

1) An analysis of molar to molar in each dental arch is known as the Total Bolton Index.
2) An analysis of canine to canine in each dental arch is known as the Anterior Bolton Index.

The total sum of the mesiodistal width of each tooth in the upper 12 teeth in ratio to the sum of the mesiodistal width of each tooth in the lower 12 teeth must be 91.3%, according to Bolton. The ideal ratio for the upper anterior 6 teeth to the lower anterior sextant is 77.2% (Ebadifar, 2013). Variations from these ratios are known as Bolton's discrepancy and the deviation of more than 2 is considered a significant discrepancy. A high ratio is an indication that mandibular teeth are larger than normal and a lower ratio is an indication that the lower teeth are smaller than normal. This analysis is particularly useful in orthodontic diagnosis to evaluate the aesthetics and the function of an occlusion. The limitation of this analysis is that discrepancies seem to be specific for gender and ethnicity.

*Soft Tissue Analyses*   Some soft tissue analyses are:

- the Holdaway line – this is a line that extends from the chin to the upper lip. Ideally, this line should bisect the nose.
- Rickett's E-plane – this line extends from the tip of the chin to the tip of the nose. Ideally, the upper lip must be slightly posterior to the line as the lower lip is positioned 2 mm anterior to the line.
- the facial plane – this line extends from the nasion to the tip of the chin. Ideally, point A must be positioned on this line and the norm angle formed between the facial plane and the Frankfort plane should be about 86 degrees.

### The Future of Cephalometrics

Computerised cephalometric analyses improve the accuracy of the diagnosis and treatment planning. The software automatically traces the landmarks and provides measurements on the digital lateral cephalometric radiograph (Figure 3.39). An example of this software program is Dolphin Imaging. The limitation of all these analyses is lack of accuracy, as true measurements are not relayed from these two-dimensional radio-

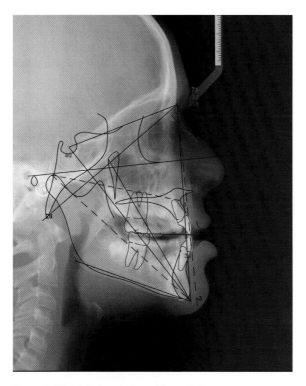

Figure 3.39  Digital cephalometric analysis.

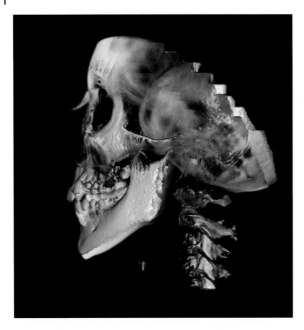

Figure 3.40 Three-dimensional radiograph. *Source*: Courtesy of Professor Ali Darendeliler.

graphs. There are software programs developed to make diagnosis and treatment planning more convenient and increase the accuracy. Three-dimensional volumes can be generated from cone beam computed tomography technologies (Harrell, 2005). Examples of some of the commonly used cone beam units are iCAT, New Tom, CB MercuRay and 3D Accuitomo.

Anatomical landmark identification is difficult on two-dimensional radiographs; hence, the accuracy of the diagnosis becomes questionable. However, with new inventions and introduction of three-dimensionally based evaluation and analysis, the precision of diagnosis and treatment will be enhanced (Figure 3.40).

### Growth Assessment Using Radiography

### Hand–Wrist Radiographs

A hand–wrist radiograph can be used to assess true biological age or skeletal maturity (Figure 3.41). This type of radiograph is extremely valuable to orthodontists as it assesses growth and maturation. It is a useful radiograph to predict the growth spurt from the bones in the wrist. This type of radiograph is usually indicated when the chronological age and the dental age do not match. The degree of ossification of the small bones in the wrist is an indication of the level of skeletal maturity. The growth of the epiphysis consists of three stages: widening, capping and fusion.

The epiphysis caps the diaphysis and eventually fuses. An indication of the growth spurt is perceived by detecting a small nodular bone adjacent to the thumb, the adductor sesamoid. Orthodontists can use various growth assessments to gain a better understanding of the maturity of the bones of the patient. The degree of ossification in the wrist provides a good assessment of skeletal age.

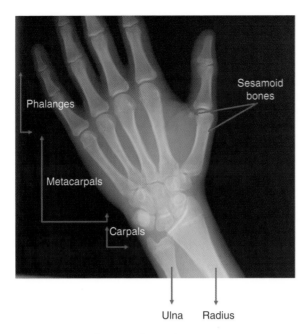

Figure 3.41 Hand–wrist radiograph.

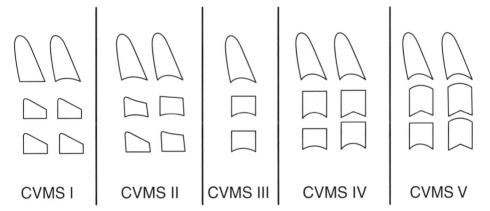

Figure 3.42 Different combinations of morphological features in the bodies of C2, C3, and C4 are presented for the new method. *Source*: Baccetti 2002. Reproduced with permission of *The Angle Orthodontist*.

**Cervical Vertebral Maturation**

Another assessment of skeletal maturity is based on the evaluation of the cervical vertebrae seen on cephalometric radiographs (Figure 3.42). Estimated growth spurt is evaluated from the level of maturation of C2 through to C4 by assessing the shape and concavity of the inferior borders of the cervical vertebrae in five maturational stages. This assessment eliminates the necessity for hand wrist radiographs. This maturational index is useful in the assessment of treatment timing for mandibular deficiencies by

Table 3.4 Summary of vertebral growth stages.

| CVSM | Definition |
| --- | --- |
| I | The lower borders of C1–C4 are flat. C3 and C4 are trapezoid in shape. The lower border of C2 can present with a concavity in some cases. The mandibular growth peak will take place at least a year after this stage and not sooner. |
| II | The lower borders of C2 and C3 present with concavities. C3 and C4 are either trapezoid or rectangular horizontal in shape. The mandibular growth peak takes place within one year after this stage. |
| III | The lower borders of C2, C3 and C4 present with concavities. C3 and C4 are no longer trapezoid but present as horizontal rectangular in shape. The mandibular growth spurt had occurred within one to two years prior to this stage. |
| Iv | The concavities in the inferior borders are present and C3 or C4 will be square in shape during this phase if not other vertebrae is still rectangular horizontal. The mandibular growth peak has taken place no later than one year before this stage. |
| V | The concavities in the lower borders remain in C2, C3 and C4. C3 or C4 may present as rectangular vertical in shape, if not the body of the other vertebrae is square. The peak in the mandibular growth has not taken place any longer than two years before this stage. |

CVSM, cervical vertebral skeletal maturation.

means of functional orthopaedics. A summary of vertebral growth stages is summarised in Table 3.4 (Baccetti et al., 2002). The study by Baccetti et al. supports that the ideal stage for functional appliance therapy for a deficient mandible is cervical vertebral maturation II as the growth peak takes place within one year after this phase.

## Treatment Planning Strategies

Treatment planning begins by developing a list of problems and goals followed by a plan on how these objectives can be achieved. The aim is to deliver the best treatment outcome possible with minimal iatrogenic adverse effects. The orthodontist carefully studies all the gathered data to create a problem list and prioritises the treatment aims, also taking into account the patient's and parent's objectives and expectations. Once a diagnosis is made and various treatment options are categorised, the next stage involves planning the appliance design, function, anchorage, biomechanics and retention. Some of the factors that influence the decision of the specialist include:

- the function and aesthetics of the malocclusion
- the psychosocial effect of the orthodontic problem and possible treatment options on the patient
- the cooperation and motivation of the patient
- the patient's general health, oral health and hygiene
- the prognosis
- the timing and complexity of the treatment.

During this phase, the orthodontist decides whether the patient will benefit from an extraction or a non-extraction based treatment. Extractions in each quadrant may or may not be the same tooth, but the objective is to have the same number of teeth extracted in each quadrant. The treatment options are discussed with the patient or guardian (if the patient is under the legal age).

The risks, benefits and costs of treatment are discussed with the patient. It is essential to ensure that the patient comprehends the processes involved as part of the treatment to make an informed consent. This allows the patient to gain a better perception of the expected outcomes and enhances compliance.

## When to refer?

Oral health therapists, dental hygienists and dental therapists need to have a clear understanding of when the patient will most benefit from an orthodontic assessment. Early intervention in some cases can use growth and development in favour of the treatment to reduce the severity of the orthodontic problem.

In contemporary orthodontics, children as young as six years can undergo orthodontic treatment. The aim of early interception is to minimise the complexity of treatment as adolescents or adults and to create adequate space for the eruption of permanent dentition. Early treatment (known as phase I) is during the mixed dentition, typically upon eruption of the permanent first molars and the incisors. It may involve partial fixed appliances and/or orthopaedic appliances that modify either the mandible or the maxilla during growth. The partial braces are referred to as '2 × 4' or '2 × 6', meaning bonding or banding of the first permanent molars and bonding of the upper four anterior teeth or the upper six anterior teeth.

Anchorage is more difficult in mixed dentition as the molars are the only source of intraoral anchorage. Achieving extraoral anchorage may be difficult in children, owing to compliance. A temporary anchorage device is not possible in children, owing to their bone porosity and the presence of permanent successors, unless it is incorporated as part an appliance to modify the jaw (see Chapter 4).

Upon completion of phase I treatment, ideal dentoalveolar modifications are made to provide sufficient space for the eruption of the permanent dentition. The second phase of treatment (phase II) in many cases is straightforward fixed appliance therapy aimed at resolving abnormalities in the occlusion, such as crowding once the permanent dentition are established. The aim of this conservative two-phase treatment is to prevent the need for extractions or orthognathic surgery by reducing the severity of the condition at an early stage. However, in cases with severe skeletal disharmony surgical correction or extractions may be inevitable in phase II.

Early intervention commences only if the orthodontist finds the patient to be a suitable candidate for this type of therapy. This judgement is most accurately made by an orthodontist; therefore, referrals are critical if abnormalities are detected during regular dental visits such as muscular imbalance, dentoalveolar or skeletal discrepancies. If the orthodontist decides that early treatment will not improve the condition or will not aid the eruption of the permanent dentition, the patient will be designated to a recall system to be monitored closely until they become a suitable candidate for orthodontic therapy. The need for orthodontic treatment is not solely based on issues associated with aesthetics or function of the occlusion. The risk of trauma and the psychosocial issues linked to the malocclusion greatly contribute to the decision for considering early treatment. A defect in an individual's physical appearance can lead to a lower self-esteem and children can suffer from discrimination as a result.

Orthodontists spend a prolonged period of time evaluating and analysing all the gathered data so that the most effective treatment can be planned for patients. They will provide all the necessary guidance and information to patients during consultations and interviews in order for an informed decision to be made. In summary, an orthodontic diagnosis is based on a problem list composed of assessments in the following areas:

- the presence of pathology
- the aesthetics and the chief complaint
- anteroposterior
- transverse
- vertical
- alignment.

## References

Alexander, R. G. *The 20 Principles of the Alexander Discipline*. Hanover Park IL: Quintessence; 2008.

Baccetti, T., Franchi, L., McNamara, J. A. Jr. An Improved Version of the Cervical Vertebral Maturation (CVM) Method for the Assessment of Mandibular Growth. *Angle Orthod*, 2002; 72(4): 316–322.

Ebadifar, A. Comparison of Bolton's ratio before and after treatment in Iranian population. *J Dent Res Dent Clin Dent Prospects*, 2013; 7(1): 30–35.

Harrell, W. E. Jr., DMD. 2005. Limitations of two-dimensional cephalometric analysis in orthodontic diagnosis and treatment planning: the future of three-dimensional analysis. *AADMRT Newsletter*, Summer 2003. Available at http://www.aadmrt.com/article-2---2003.html (accessed 6 April 2017).

Kravitz, D., Groth, C., Jones, P. et al. Intraoral digital scanners. *J Clin Orthod*, 2014; 48(6): 337–347.

McDonald, F. *Diagnosis of the Orthodontic Patient*. Oxford: Oxford University Press; 1998.

Mitchell, L. *An Introduction to Orthodontics*. 3rd ed. Oxford: Oxford University Press; 2007.

Moore, T, Southard, K. A., Casko, C. S., et al. Buccal corridors and smile esthetics. *Am J Orthod Dentofacial Orthop*, 2005; 127(2): 208–213.

Nandini, V. V. Alginate impressions: A practical perspective. *J Conserv Dent*, 2008; 11(1): 37–41.

Wassell, R. W., Barker, D., Walls, A. W. Crowns and other extra-coronal restorations: impression materials and technique. *Br Dent J*, 2002; 192(12): 679–690.

## Further Reading

Ackerman, M. B., Ackerman, J. L. Smile analysis and design in the digital era. *J Clin Orthod*, 36(4): 221–236.

Ahmad, I. Digital dental photography. Part 1: an overview. *Br Dent J*, 2009; 206: 403–407.

Bishara, S. E. *Textbook of Orthodontics*. Philadelphia, PA: W.B. Saunders; 2001.

Brand, R. W., Isselhard, D. E. *Anatomy of Orofacial Structures: A comprehensive approach*. 7th ed. St Louis, MO: Elsevier Mosby.

Burstone, C. J., Marcotte, M. E. *Problem Solving in Orthodontics: Goal-Oriented Treatment Strategies*. Hanover Park, IL: Quintessence; 2000.

Chiego, D. J. *Essentials of Oral Histology and Embryology: A clinical approach*. 4th ed. St Louis, MO: Elsevier Mosby; 2014.

Downs, W. B. Analysis of the dentofacial profile. *Angle Orthod*, 1956; 26(4): 191–212.

Foster, T. D. *A Textbook of Orthodontics*. 3rd ed. Oxford: Blackwell Scientific; 1990.

Goose, D. H., Appleton, D. G. *Human Dentofacial Growth*. Oxford: Pergamon Press; 1982.

Kravitz, N. D., Groth, C., Jones, P. E., et al. Intraoral digital scanners. *J Clin Orthod*, 2014; 48(6): 337–347.

Nayar, S., Mahadevan, R. A paradigm shift in the concept for making dental impressions. *J Pharm Bioallied Sci*, 2015; 7(Suppl 1): S213–215.

Ooë, T. *Human Tooth and Dental Arch Development*. Tokyo: Ishiyaku Publishers; 1981.

Park, J. U., Baik, S. H. Classification of angle class III malocclusion and its treatment modalities. *Int J Adult Orthod*, 2001; 16(1): 19–29.

Ranly, D. M. (ed.) *A Synopsis of Craniofacial Growth*. 2nd ed. Norwalk, CT: Appleton and Lange; 1990.

Roberts-Harry, D., Sandy, J. Orthodontics. Part 2: Patient assessment and examination. *Br Dent J*, 2003; 195: 489–493.

Stewart, R. F., Edgar, H., Tatlock, C., et al. Developing a standardized cephalometric vocabulary: choices and possible strategies. *J Dent Educ*, 2008; 72(9): 989–997.

Welbury, R. R., Duggal, M. S., Hosey, M. T. *Paediatric Dentistry*. 4th ed. Oxford: Oxford University Press; 2012.

Wiet, G. J. Biavati, M. J., Rocha-Worley, G. Reconstructive surgery for cleft palate treatment and management. Medscape, 17 August 2015. Available at http://emedicine.medscape.com/article/878062-treatment (accessed 7 April 2017).

## Self-Evaluation

1   Which of the following data must be collected at the initial consultation?
     **A** Medical history.
     **B** Dental history.
     **C** Family and social history.
     **D** All the above (a–c).

2   Which radiograph is most suitable to aid an orthodontic diagnosis?
     **A** Lateral cephalometrics.
     **B** Occlusal radiographs.
     **C** Periapical radiographs.
     **D** Bite wings.

3   What is the term given to protrusion of both the maxilla and the mandible alveolar processes?
     **A** Prognathic.
     **B** Retrognathic.
     **C** Bimaxillary.
     **D** Mesognathic.

4 Why is obtaining medical and dental history a crucial aspect of treatment planning?
   A Better patient management.
   B Aids in diagnosis.
   C Medico-legal documents.
   D Aids in prevention and management of medical emergencies.
   E All of the above (a–d).

5 In which category of impression material does alginate belong to?
   A Non-elastic.
   B Elastic.
   C Addition cured silicone.
   D Hydrocolloid.
   E b and d.

6 How does class I molar occlusion present?
   A Mesiobuccal cusp of the upper first permanent molar occludes on the mesiobuccal groove of the lower second permanent molar.
   B Mesiobuccal cusp of the upper first permanent molar occludes mesial to the mesiobuccal groove of the lower first permanent molar.
   C Mesiobuccal cusp of the upper second permanent molar occludes on the mesiobuccal groove of the lower second permanent molar.
   D Mesiobuccal cusp of the upper first permanent molar occludes on the mesiobuccal groove of the lower first permanent molar.

7 What is imbibition of a dental impression?
   A Shrinkage of the material.
   B Tear in the material.
   C Swelling due to excessive water.
   D Evaporation of water from the material.

8 Which of the following is considered as norm according to the anteroposterior radiographic diagnosis?
   A SNA greater than 82 degrees.
   B SNB less than 80 degrees.
   C ANB 2 degrees.
   D ANB 7 degrees.

9 Which radiograph aids in assessment of the growth spurt?
   A Hand–wrist radiograph only.
   B Orthopantomogram and cephalometric radiograph.
   C Cephalometric radiograph and hand–wrist radiograph.
   D Occlusal radiographs.

10 Which of the following facial profiles is typically seen in class III skeletal patterns?
   A A convex profile due to the mandible.
   B A convex profile due to the maxilla.
   C A concave profile.
   D A straight profile.

# 4

# Biomechanics and Treatment Principles

The treatment modality for each individual with an orthodontic or an orthognathic problem will vary greatly, depending on several factors. Every malocclusion and skeletal discrepancy cannot be treated using the same treatment protocol. Although the biomechanics are the same, they are used in various ways. This chapter focuses on the fundamentals of tooth movement and provides a summary of anchorage.

## Biomechanics

Orthodontic biomechanics is the study of the biological systems involved in tooth movement. Control of orthodontic treatment is achieved by understanding the reactions of dental and facial structures to orthodontic forces. Thus, for better decision making and efficiency of care, it is essential to have knowledge of the factors governing tooth movement.

## The Mechanics of Tooth Movement

### Force, Moment, Couple

Physical properties are categorised as scalars or vectors. Scalars do not have a direction but do have a definite magnitude; for example, weight. Vectors have both magnitude and direction; for example, force. The force applied to teeth with a tendency to cause rotation is known as the moment of force. The size of this component of force is mathematically calculated by multiplying the magnitude of the applied force by the perpendicular distance between the point of application and the centre of resistance (Gill, 2008). This is important in orthodontics as force is applied to the crown of a tooth since it cannot be directly applied to the centre of resistance located on the root. Consequently, rotation of the tooth occurs (Figure 4.1).

The term 'couple' is given to two parallel forces of the same magnitude in opposing directions to rotate a tooth. The size of this component of force is calculated by multiplying the magnitude of applied forces by the distance between them. To describe a moment or couple, the term torque is used in orthodontics (Gill, 2008).

*Orthodontics for Dental Hygienists and Dental Therapists*, First Edition. Tina Raked.
© 2018 John Wiley & Sons Ltd. Published 2018 by John Wiley & Sons Ltd.
Companion website: www.wiley.com/go/raked/orthodontics_dental_hygienists

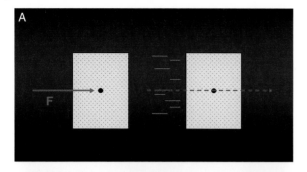

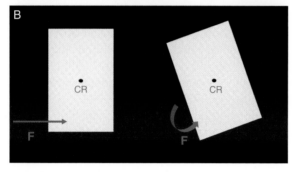

Figure 4.1 Force: A) Force (F) must be applied directly to the centre of resistance (CR) of an object to move it in the direction of the force. B) If force (F) does not pass through the centre of resistance (CR), rotation occurs. *Source*: Courtesy of Professor Ali Darendeliler.

### Centre of Resistance, Centre of Rotation

The centre of resistance is the point of resistance to movement. This point is usually located in the middle of an object in a homogenous environment (Figure 4.1A). In a heterogeneous environment, the centre of resistance is towards the denser side (Figure 4.2). The root of the tooth is embedded in bone; therefore, the centre of gravity or point of balance of the tooth is more apically located due to bone density (Figure 4.3). On single rooted teeth, the centre of resistance is half way between the root apex and the alveolar bone crest. In a multi-rooted tooth, the centre of resistance is one to two millimetres apical to the furcation. The centre of resistance is influenced by length of the root and height of the alveolar crest. Longer roots have a lower centre of resistance. As bone loss increases, the centre of resistance becomes located further apically. This is because the density of the environment greatly affects the centre of resistance. Bodily movement occurs as the force passes through the centre of resistance. If force does not pass through the centre of resistance, tipping results.

The centre of rotation is the rotation of a body from its original position (Figure 4.4). Tooth movement does not alter the centre of resistance; however, the centre of rotation varies depending on the type of tooth movement; for example, the centre of rotation lies at the apex for tilting the crown of the tooth while the centre of rotation lies at infinity if the crown and the root are moved as a unit.

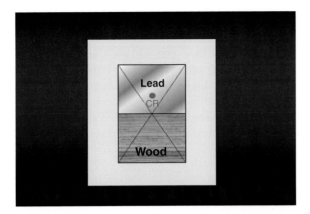

Figure 4.2 The centre of resistance (CR) is towards the denser side and not in the centre of the object. *Source*: Courtesy of Professor Ali Darendeliler.

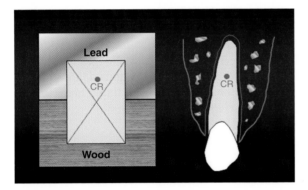

Figure 4.3 The tooth is embedded in bone, therefore the centre of resistance (CR) is not in the centre of the tooth. As the bone is more dense, the centre of resistance is located further apically. *Source*: Courtesy of Professor Ali Darendeliler.

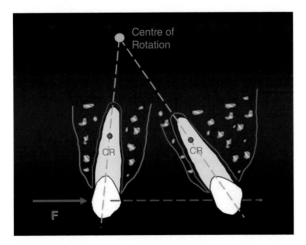

Figure 4.4 Centre of rotation. *Source*: Courtesy of Professor Ali Darendeliler.

## The Biology of Tooth Movement

Collagenous supporting fibres called periodontal ligaments anchor the tooth in the bony socket by maintaining a strong attachment between the alveolar bone, gingiva and the root cementum. Tooth movement is made possible with the presence of periodontal ligaments and their cellular elements, such as undifferentiated mesenchymal cells and tissue fluid in the periodontal ligament space. There are two theories supporting the biological control of tooth movement, the bioelectric theory and the pressure tension theory.

### Bioelectric Theory

The electricity travelling through the periodontal ligaments is piezoelectric. The piezo-electricity initiates a rapid response but, regardless of the force sustainability, it decays or dies away quickly to zero. Another characteristic is reaching equilibrium upon release of force. It is believed that piezoelectric responses are caused by the bending of the alveolar bone. The flex of the bone causes a localised production of prostaglandins, which facilitates tooth movement. This theory supports the fact that tooth movement is carried out by stress on the alveolar bone rather than the periodontal ligaments. Some studies suggest that forces stress the bone, precipitating electrical charges in response to the deformities. Negative polarity on the concavities results in bone deposition and positive polarity of the convex surfaces of the bone results in resorption. These bioelectric variances lead to bone remodelling (Proffit, 2007).

### Pressure Tension Theory

The shock of the force is absorbed within the periodontal ligament space and a cascade of chemical reactions occurs to make tooth movement possible (Figure 4.5). The direction of the force is the decisive factor for which part of the supporting structures of the tooth undergo pressure or tension. When force is applied to teeth, the periodontal ligament undergoes pressure on the side towards the movement and tension on the opposite side away from the movement. The side with compression and pressure undergoes resorption by bone resorptive cells (osteoclasts) as the alveolar bone deforms and blood supply to the area increases, resulting in mobilisation of cells such as osteoclasts. On the tension side, an increased blood flow is evident to the area owing to stretching of the ligaments.

In response to force, osteoblasts produce prostaglandin $E_2$ and leukotrienes, owing to the deformities developed in the periodontal ligaments and the bone. These cells are responsive to mechanical loading and are found in areas of inflammation. Prostaglandin $E_2$ is a mediator in bone resorption and leukotrienes increase intracellular messengers to the site. Examples of these intracellular messengers are interleukin-1 and macrophage colony-stimulating factor (MCSF). Interleukin-1, produced by osteoblasts and macrophages, stimulates bone resorption and inhibit bone formation by increasing prostaglandin synthesis. MCSF is also produced by osteoblasts to coordinate osteoclasts proliferation and differentiation. As these messengers are recruited to the site, an increased production of osteoblasts and receptor activator of nuclear factor kappa-B ligand (RANKL) is evident. RANKL is secreted by osteoblasts as a stimulating factor for differentiation, fusion and activation of osteoclastic cells. This factor is essential in

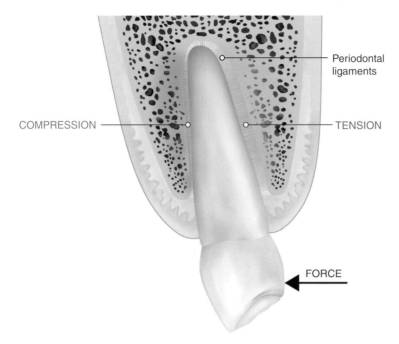

Figure 4.5 Tension and compression.

osteoclast survival. As a result of these events, macrophages produce more interleukin-1, leading to an increased level of RANKL. RANKL and MCSF attract additional blood monocytes to the site. The blood monocytes fuse to form osteoclasts and become activated by RANKL.

Osteoid is exposed to allow access to the underlying mineralised bone. Osteoid is a newly formed layer of bone as a result of osteoblastic activity; it matures within about ten days (Foster, 1990). Matrix metalloproteinases are produced by osteoblasts to break down the osteoid and permit access to the underlying mature bone. Osteoclasts are recruited to the site and secrete hydrogen ions into the matrix. These ions soften the hydroxyapatite crystals and degrade the extracellular matrix with proteases. These events lead to bone resorption. The activity of bone resorptive cells are inhibited by the production of enzymes and cytokines. Bone resorption is strictly controlled by osteoblasts, as it produces cells such as osteoprotegerin to block the effect of RANKL. Osteoblasts are vital in the coordination of bone homeostasis.

On the side with tension, a series of events takes place leading to bone formation. Owing to a tensile force, the osteoblasts flatten and allow access to osteoid. The periodontal ligaments respond to these changes by increasing the levels of specific secondary messengers (extracellular signal-regulated kinase, ERK). ERK increases the activity of osteoblasts, and thus bone formation, by inducing expression of runt-related transcription factor 2 (RUNX2). The fibroblasts of periodontal ligament differentiate into osteoblasts induced by RUNX-2 (Mitchell, 2001).

These cascades of events lead to bone remodelling, which is responsible for tooth movement. These alterations occur for the bone to accommodate movement of the bony socket from one place to another and to make orthodontic tooth movement possible.

## Orthodontic Forces

Light continuous forces permit tooth movement as hyperaemia (increased blood flow) recruits osteoblasts and osteoclasts to the site, causing frontal resorption. This type of resorption takes place in the inner wall of the alveolar bone between the root and the lamina dura. Constant gentle forces resorb the bone on the side of the socket, which undergoes pressure as bone deposition takes place on the side of the socket with tension. The tensile pressure increases vascularity and osteoid develops at the site, which is more resistant to resorption in comparison with alveolar bone.

Strong continuous forces result in ischaemia (inadequate blood flow) of the periodontal ligaments due to extreme compression and pressure. This leads to undermining resorption of the socket wall. Excessive heavy forces crush and occlude the periodontal ligaments, resulting in tissue necrosis (cell death). This may lead to unwanted tooth resorption or ankylosis (the fusion of tooth and bone). Ankylosis occurs as the tooth contacts the bone from compression of the ligaments.

Heavy forces cause hyalinisation of the periodontal ligaments. Since hyaline tissue degenerates, the tissues appears translucent and smooth as they lose their cellular elements. This zone disappears with resorption by osteoclasts. During compression, cells from periphery tissues can also invade the hyalinised tissue and obliterate the layer.

The force magnitude and duration is responsible for the type of resorption that takes place. Frontal resorption (Figure 4.6) is ideal for tooth movement and less painful for the patient, although undermining resorption (Figure 4.7) might occur at some stages throughout the treatment, irrespective of the care given to avoid it. It is extremely important to understand these processes to detect abnormalities during treatment at an

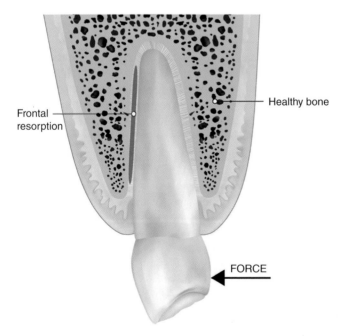

**Figure 4.6** Frontal resorption.

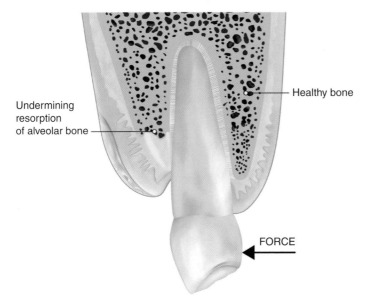

Undermining resorption of alveolar bone

Healthy bone

FORCE

Figure 4.7 Undermining resorption.

early stage. Clinically, moderate mobility is considered a normal part of orthodontic treatment as the tooth socket relocates. However, excessive mobility occurs as teeth move in a traumatic occlusion and as persistent heavy forces cause exorbitant undermining resorption. During regular appointments, it is crucial to assess the degree of mobility and notify the orthodontist if excessive mobility is detected. Typically, relieving the tooth of the traumatic occlusion and reducing the forces will allow better blood flow to the compressed areas, allowing the ligaments to reattach firmly.

Studies suggest that favourable forces are lower than capillary blood pressure, which is 32 mmHg. The dental pulp has a transient response to initiation of orthodontic appliances, causing mild pulpitis. However, as discussed previously, uncontrolled excessive forces can cause pulpal necrosis. If a tooth presents with an existing non-vital pulp, orthodontic movement is feasible in the absence of periapical pathology.

### Types of Tooth movement

There are different types of movement:

- Tipping: the tilting of the tooth away from the force.
  The closer the force to the occlusal or incisal surfaces, the closer the centre of rotation to the apex of the tooth. There are two types of tipping: controlled and uncontrolled. Controlled tipping is movement of the crown in the same direction as the force while the root remains unaffected or has minimal movement. The centre of rotation lies at the apex. Uncontrolled tipping occurs when the crown moves in the same direction as the force and the root moves in an opposite direction. The centre of rotation lies close to the centre of resistance. Force for tipping should not exceed 50 g.
- Translation (bodily movement): the crown and the root move in the same direction as the force.

To avoid tilting of the tooth, it is essential to apply the force on a wider area of the crown. The periodontal ligament is loaded evenly with this type of movement. The force level for translation is about 50–120 g.

- Rotation: the rotating of the tooth in its sockets is known as a rotational movement. This movement occurs where forces are applied to opposite sides of the tooth. It is highly susceptible to relapse, owing to stretching of the gingival fibres. The force needed for rotational tooth movement is about 35–60 g. Tipping can occur because of excessive compression of the periodontal ligaments.
- Torque: the root moves in the same direction as the force as the crown remains unaffected or has minimal movement.
  This is the opposite of tipping. The centre of rotation lies towards the occlusal surfaces. The force level is about 50–100 g.
- Vertical movements: require bodily movement of the tooth classified as extrusion and intrusion.
  Extrusion occurs as the tooth is pushed out of the socket. This movement requires more tension than pressure as bone is deposited at the root apex. Intrusion occurs as the tooth is pushed further into the socket. This type of movement requires substantial resorption at the root apex as the supporting structures undergo pressure and not tension. The roots are susceptible to shortening due to resorption. The force levels for extrusion is about 35–60 g and intrusion requires about 10–20 g of force.

There are certain prescribed medications that suppress tooth movement. Bisphosphonates are indicated for treatment of osteoporosis. Tooth movement is delayed by this medication as it inhibits the osteoclastic cells to reduce bone resorption. Corticosteroids and nonsteroidal anti-inflammatory drugs are also examples of medications that impede rapid tooth movement. These medications are prostaglandin inhibitors and, as mentioned previously, prostaglandin E2 plays a major role in the chemical cascade that makes tooth movement possible (Arias and Marquez-Orozco, 2006).

## Anchorage

Newton's third law states that for every action, there is an equal and opposite reaction. Newton's third law of attraction also applies to tooth movement. The resistance to unintended orthodontic movement is termed 'anchorage'. When orthodontists intend to move certain teeth, other teeth will move if they are in contact with the appliance. The teeth that require minimal movement become anchor units for the movement of other teeth. This is achieved by applying minimal force to the periodontal ligaments of the teeth in the anchor unit to prevent displacement. The occurrence of unwanted tooth movement or displacement is termed 'loss of anchorage'. This occurs as the teeth in the anchor unit move more than anticipated. Causes of anchorage loss include:

- poor patient compliance
- ill-fitting appliances
- obstructions in the path of tooth movement
- insufficient anchorage for the planned orthodontic movement.

Some common clinical findings of anchorage loss are:

- proclined anterior teeth resulting in an increased overjet
- excessive spacing
- inclination of the teeth in the anchor unit
- poor appliance fit.

If the anchor unit is displaced intentionally, this is termed slipped, blown or burn anchorage. A typical example of this displacement is closure of the extraction spaces by moving the molars anteriorly.

Orthodontists plan anchorage into their treatment prior to commencement of treatment. Several factors influence the necessity for different types of anchorage. The number of teeth, distance and type of movement contribute to the degree of anchorage required; for example, higher anchorage is indicated if teeth have to be moved a greater distance and if more teeth are to be moved. Bodily movements require more anchorage than tipping. The degree of anchorage required is categorised as maximum anchorage, moderate anchorage and mild anchorage:

- Maximum anchorage: anchorage maintenance and monitoring is critical as minimal anchorage can be lost.
- Moderate anchorage: anchorage is important but not critical.
- Minimum anchorage: loss of anchorage can be desirable for an optimum treatment outcome.

### Anchorage Site

Sources of anchorage can be teeth, musculature, bone or implants. The anchorage site is classified as extraoral and intraoral. Extraoral anchorage sources can be occipital, cervical and facial (Figure 4.8). A disadvantage of extraoral anchorage is that it requires significant patient compliance for achieving optimal results. Intra oral anchorage is further classified as intra-maxillary (within the same dental arch) or inter-maxillary (distributed between opposite arches).

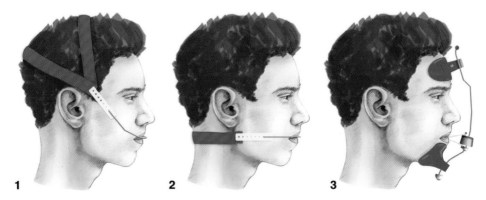

Figure 4.8 Extraoral appliances used as anchorage (to see how these appliances move teeth please refer to chapters 7 and 8). 1) Cranium: (occipital/parietal anchorage) headgears with a face bow to restrict maxillary growth or distalise the upper arch. 2) Cervical: back of the neck as anchorage using a cervical head gear/neck strap. 3) Facial: face masks use frontal bone and the mandibular symphysis as anchorage during treatment. Face masks are also known as reverse head gears.

Anchorage had been also classified as:

- Simple/primary: resistance to tipping movements using one tooth.
- Compound: achieving movement by using two or a group of teeth as anchorage.
- Reinforced: using non-dental sites for additional source of anchorage such as muscles.
- Stationary: resistance to translation or bodily movement of the teeth. An example of stationary anchorage is retraction of the maxillary incisors using maxillary molars as anchorage. It is termed stationary as the teeth in the anchor unit are not free to move.
- Reciprocal: movement of teeth in equal and opposite directions (equal distribution of force within the periodontal ligament). Closing the anterior diastema is an example of this type of anchorage.

### Intermaxillary Anchorage

Intermaxillary anchorage uses opposing arches as anchor units to achieve the desired shifts in the alveolar bone of the maxilla or mandible. Elastic wear does not alter basal bone but shifts the alveolus to the desired position depending on the pattern of elastic wear. Usually, elastics are worn in combination with stronger wires that can withstand the force. Initial arch wires and elastic wear provide minimal torque control and can cause unwanted tipping (Alexander, 2008). Some of the most common patterns of elastic wear are listed in Table 4.1 and illustrated in Figure 4.9. Elastics are only worn in the permanent dentition. The primary objective of the elastic wear is to coordinate dental arches. Depending on what the orthodontist is trying to achieve, a combination of elastics can be worn. There are variations to these patterns, depending on what the specialist orthodontist is trying to achieve. It is therefore critical to confirm what teeth are included in the elastic wear before giving patient the instructions.

### Intramaxillary Anchorage

Intramaxillary anchorage achieves tooth movement with anchorage units in the same arch (Figure 4.10).

### Temporary Anchorage Devices

Skeletal anchorage has become a popular solution that is proven to provide high success in clinical practice. Skeletal anchorage systems use implants with various nomenclature such as (Ludwig et al., 2008):

- pins
- micro-implants
- mini-implants
- mini-screws
- temporary anchorage devices.

In contemporary orthodontics, temporary anchorage devices are becoming a popular source of intraoral anchorage (Figure 4.11). Such devices can provide adequate anchorage for space closures without retruding the anterior segment, thus preventing

Table 4.1 Some common elastic patterns.

| Elastic Pattern | Configuration | Movement Achieved | Key[a] |
|---|---|---|---|
| Class I (type of intramaxillary anchorage) | First molars to canine or posts/hooks on arch wires | This is typically used for extraction space closure | 1 |
| Class II | Upper canine to lower first molar | Dental class II correction. Retraction of the upper anterior segment | 2 |
| Class II triangle | Upper canine, lower first premolar to lower first molar | Corrects class II and the vertical overlap | 3 |
| Class III | Upper first molar to lower canine | Dental class III correction. Retraction of the lower anterior segment as it prevents lower incisor flaring. | 4 |
| Class III triangle | Upper first molar, upper first premolar to lower canine | Corrects class III and the vertical overlap | 5 |
| Delta or triangle | Upper canine to lower canine and lower first premolar | Increase overbite and corrects canine interdigitation | 6 |
| Anterior cross elastic | From the upper canine to the lower canine in the opposite quadrant. This diagonal anterior elastic has variations depending on whether the midline shift correction is to the left or right. | Midline shift correction | 7 |
| Posterior cross elastic | Palatal of one or more upper teeth to the buccal of one or more lower teeth | Correction of posterior cross bite. | 8 |
| Box elastic | Typically involves two or more teeth in the upper and two or more teeth in the lower arch | Correction of open bite. Allows extrusion of upper and lower teeth. Box elastics can be anterior or posterior. It aids in mandibular arch levelling and provides vertical correction. | 9, 10 |

[a] Corresponding number in Figure 4.9.

lip support deficiency. These devices allow the uprighting of the molars without unwanted extrusion or disturbances to the surrounding teeth (McGuire et al., 2006). They are manufactured in numerous designs and sizes to accommodate for various mucosal thicknesses. Temporary anchorage devices are non-toxic, biocompatible and may be composed of titanium, titanium alloys or titanium-coated stainless steel. An essential property of the material used is to withstand orthodontic loading to enable the anchorage necessary for effective results. Mini-screw implants can be used as direct or indirect anchorage (Figure 4.13). For direct anchorage, auxiliaries such as elastics or springs are directly connected to the implant to provide adequate skeletal anchorage (Figure 4.12). For indirect anchorage, a segmented wire is incorporated with the mini-screw to provide a supporting structure and prevent unintended tooth movement.

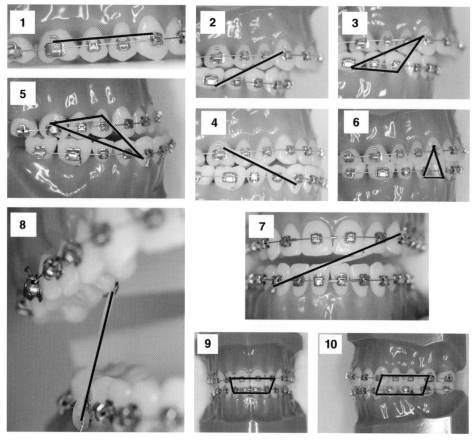

Figure 4.9 Some common elastic patterns. 1) Class I. 2) Class II. 3) Class II triangle. 4) Class III. 5) Class III triangle. 6) Delta. 7) Anterior cross elastic. 8) Posterior cross elastic. 9) Anterior box elastic. 10) Posterior box elastic.

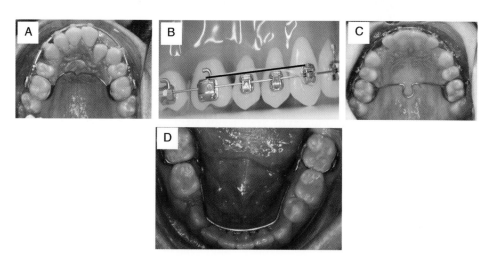

Figure 4.10 Examples of intramaxillary anchorage. A) Nance with an acrylic button. B) Class I mechanics. C) Transpalatal arch. D) Lower lingual holding arch.

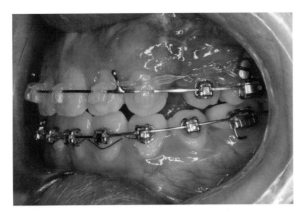

Figure 4.11 Intramaxillary anchorage used to retract the anterior segment and close extraction spaces.

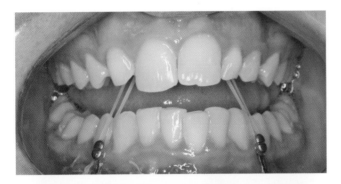

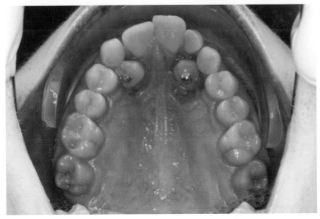

Figure 4.12 Skeletal plates used as a source of anchorage in combination with elastic wear to extrude the ectopic canines.

### Indications

Mini-screws are extremely effective for:

- mesial and distal translations with restrictions, such as distalising molars
- intrusion of overerupted teeth
- extrusion and uprighting molars
- space closures
- reduce occlusal plane cants.

### Application

These mini-screw implants are drilled into the medullary and cortical bone. There are two types of mini-screws: self-tapping (recommended for the lower jaw) and self-drilling (recommended for the upper jaw). The major difference between the two types is the mode of insertion (Figure 4.13). Self-tapping screws require a pilot drill to remove

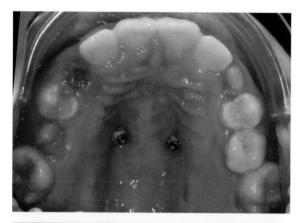

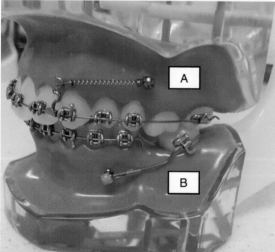

Figure 4.13 Temporary anchorage devices inserted in the palatal region. A) directly loaded. B) Indirectly located.

osseous tissue before insertion to create space for the mass in the bone. The mini-screw is placed in the bone with a hand screwdriver. Self-drilling does not require the use of a pilot drill as the cutting edge of the screw penetrates the bone. This procedure takes place under local anaesthetic. Before insertion, radiographs and clinical examinations are carried out by the specialist to confirm the position of the mini-screw.

Preparation may slightly vary between practitioners. A guideline for delivery of the screw is summarised below (Ballard et al., 2007):

- Prepare and plan by taking radiographs and carrying out a through clinical examination.
- Rinse the oral cavity with chlorhexidine to reduce bacterial flora.
- Apply topical anaesthesia.
- Apply local anaesthesia.
- Select the type of screw (determine the length and diameter).
- Take a periapical radiograph to detect the insertion point.
- Perforate the gingiva with the screw or punch with specific instruments, if needed by the specialist.
- Prepare the bone with or without pilot drill, depending on the screw design and bone quality.
- Insert the screw.
- Specialists may take a periapical radiograph to ensure correct positioning.
- Load immediately.

To enhance the stability of the screw, orthodontists will ensure that there is sufficient osseous density, cortical thickness and adequate distance between the roots of the teeth.

Oral hygiene is crucial for a successful treatment outcome as plaque accumulation leads to peri-implantitis and failure of the mini screws. The patient must be advised to keep the implants clean and free of plaque using interdental brushes for better access.

### Screw Removal

Removal of the mini-screw can take place with or without local anaesthesia. Since the mini-screws are not osseointegrated, simply unscrewing the implant will suffice. Wound healing of the area takes place within a few days after removal. The area must be kept free of plaque.

### Contraindications

Systemic contraindications for implant therapy are:

- bleeding disorders
- diabetes mellitus
- bone metabolic disorders
- titanium allergy
- anti-coagulant treatment
- immune deficiency disorders.

Local contraindicating factors include:

- xerostomia
- poor oral hygiene

- smoking
- presence of pathology
- insufficient bone quality.

### Factors Affecting Anchorage

Factors affecting anchorage include:

- root morphology
- root surface area
- the number of roots
- direction of force
- type of tooth movement and duration
- bone density
- growth.

Multi-roots, longer roots and roots with a triangular cross-section require less anchorage, as they offer a degree of resistance to tooth movement. Bodily movements require more anchorage than tipping.

## References

Alexander, R. G. *The 20 Principles of the Alexander Discipline.* Hanover Park IL: Quintessence; 2008.

Arias, O. R., Marquez-Orozco, M. C. Aspirin, acetaminophen, and ibuprofen: Their effects on orthodontic tooth movement. *Am J Orthod Dentofacial Orthop*, 2006; 130(3): 364–370.

Ballard, D., Darendeliler, A., Vickers, D., et al. Orthodontics and mini-screws. *Brighter Futures*, 2007; (3): 1–4. Available at https://2-aso.cdn.aspedia.net/sites/default/files/uploaded-content/field_f_content_file/orthodontics_and_mini-screws.pdf (accessed 7 April 2017).

Foster, T. D. *A Textbook of Orthodontics.* 3rd ed. Oxford: Blackwell Scientific; 1990.

Gill D. S. *Orthodontics at a Glance.* Oxford: Wiley-Blackwell Publishing; 2008.

Ludwig, B., Baumgaertel, S., Bowman, J. (eds). *Mini-Implants in Orthodontics. Innovative Anchorage Concept.* Hanover Park, IL: Quintessence.

Mitchell, L. *An Introduction to Orthodontics.* 3rd ed. Oxford: Oxford University Press; 2007.

Proffit, W. R., Fields, H. W., Sarver, D. M. *Contemporary Orthodontics.* 5th ed. St Louis, MO: Mosby Elsevier; 2012.

## Further Reading

Bishara, S. E. *Textbook of Orthodontics.* Philadelphia, PA: W.B. Saunders; 2001.

Chin, M. Y., Sandham, A., de Vries, J., et al. Biofilm formation on surface characterized micro-implants for skeletal anchorage in orthodontics. *Biomaterials*, 2007; 28(11): 2032–2040.

Cope, J. B. Temporary anchorage devices in orthodontics: A paradigm shift. *Semin Orthod*, 2005; 11: 3–9.

Cornelis, M. A., Scheffler, N. R., De Clerck, H. J., et al. Systematic review of the experimental use of temporary skeletal anchorage devices in orthodontics. *Am J Orthod Dentofacial Orthop*, 2007; 131(4 Suppl): S52–S58.

Higuchi, K. W., Slack, J. M. The use of Titanium fixtures for intraoral anchorage to facilitate orthodontic tooth movement. *Int J Oral Maxillofac implants*, 1991; 6(3): 338–344.

McGuire, M. K., Scheyer, E. T., Gallerano, R. L. Temporary anchorage devices for tooth movement: a review and case reports. *J Periodontol*, 2006; 77(10): 1613–1624.

## Self-Evaluation

1 What is the difference between scalars and vectors?
   **A** Scalars have a definite magnitude; vectors have both a definite direction and a magnitude.
   **B** Vectors have a definite direction while scalars have a definite magnitude.
   **C** Scalars and vectors both have a definite magnitude but scalars have a definite direction as well.

2 Where is the centre of resistance located on single-rooted teeth?
   **A** At the apex of the root.
   **B** Half way between the root apex and the alveolar bone crest.
   **C** On the cementoenamel junction.

3 What makes tooth movement possible?
   **A** Remodelling of the alveolar bone caused by a cascade of reactions due to osteoblasts and osteoclasts.
   **B** Tension of the periodontal ligaments on the side opposite to the force and pressure of the periodontal ligaments on the side of movement.
   **C** Both of the above (a and b).

4 What type of forces are ideal for tooth movement?
   **A** Heavy continuous forces.
   **B** Light continuous forces.
   **C** Heavy intermittent forces.

5 What is frontal resorption?
   **A** Resorption in the inner wall of the alveolar bone due to light continuous forces.
   **B** Hyalinisation of the periodontal ligaments.
   **C** Resorption of the alveolar bone due to heavy continuous forces.

6 What is the name given to the type of tooth movement that results in minimal movement of the crown but movement of the root in the same direction as the force?
   **A** Translation.
   **B** Torque.
   **C** Extrusion.

7  What is reciprocal anchorage?
  **A** Resistance to bodily movement.
  **B** Movement of the teeth in equal and opposite directions.
  **C** Resistance to tipping movements.

8  Temporary anchorage devices are contraindicated in patients with bleeding disorders.
  **A** True.
  **B** False.

9  What are some of the advantages of temporary anchorage devices?
  **A** They can provide anchorage for some space closure cases without resulting in retrusion of the anterior segment.
  **B** Uprighting of molars without unwanted extrusion or disturbance to surrounding teeth.
  **C** Both of the above (a and b).

10  What factors affect the degree of anchorage needed?
  **A** The number of teeth that need to be moved.
  **B** The distance and type of movement.
  **C** Both of the above (a and b).

5

# Fixed Appliances and Orthodontic Instruments

Orthodontic appliances that are bonded to teeth and cannot be removed by the patient are termed 'fixed appliances'. Depending on the type and design, fixed appliances can be used for anchorage, correction of some skeletal or jaw discrepancies and for the treatment of dental irregularities. Examples of some of the fixed appliances for jaw corrections are the Herbst®, Forsus™ or palatal expanders that are discussed further in Chapters 6, 7 and 8. Braces are fixed appliances used for treating dental misalignment and disharmony. The focus of this chapter is on braces, and provides a brief summary of the history of braces and a review of some of the most commonly used instruments and ligatures. Precise tooth movement is carried out with the use of fixed appliances. Successful treatment outcomes are achieved with braces in reduction of overbite, multiple tooth movement, relief of crowding, space closures, correction of rotations and more.

## Fixed Appliances

The interaction between the metal attachments on the tooth called bracket and the arch wire determines the direction of the movement. There is an extensive variety of materials and designs for brackets and arch wires. Wires are classified according to their cross-section as either round or rectangular (Figure 5.1). Interactions between the round wire and the bracket slot allows tipping in buccolingual directions with a degree of mesiodistal tipping and rotational positioning. Rectangular wires are used after a period of using arch wires with a round cross-section to gain better control of the tooth movement. The rectangular wires completely engage in the bracket slot thus permit bodily tooth movements.

Unlike removable appliances, fixed appliances allow several tooth movements such as rotations, extrusion, intrusion, uprighting and torque. The difference between up righting the roots and torque is the direction of root movement. Uprighting is made possible by mesiodistal movements along the length of the arch wire. Torque is made possible by labiolingual movements with right-angle bends on the arch wire. Specific movement and torque is made with various types of bends categorised as first-order, second-order and third-order bend. The orthodontist will use specific pliers to bend stainless steel or beta-titanium wires to complete final root and crown adjustments. Most bracket systems have prescribed palatal root torque within the bracket slot. Once engaged with a

*Orthodontics for Dental Hygienists and Dental Therapists*, First Edition. Tina Raked.
© 2018 John Wiley & Sons Ltd. Published 2018 by John Wiley & Sons Ltd.
Companion website: www.wiley.com/go/raked/orthodontics_dental_hygienists

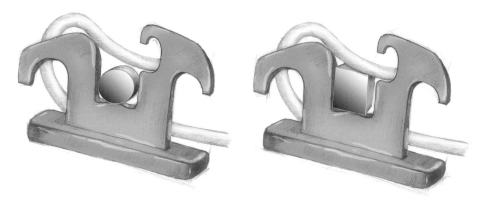

Figure 5.1 A cross-section showing the difference between a round and a rectangular arch wire in a bracket slot.

rectangular arch wire, the root moves palatally and the crown moves labially. In some instances, orthodontists may bond a bracket upside down to achieve the opposite effect and move the root labially as the crown moves palatally.

### Evolution of Bracket Systems

In the 17th century, a French dentist, Pierre Fauchard (known as the father of orthodontics) introduced orthodontics with an arch-shaped metal band. This introduction to orthodontics was suitable for tipping teeth with minimal rotational control. In the 20th century, Edward Hartley Angle (known as the father of modern orthodontics) introduced the Edgewise appliance after devising the classification of malocclusion (see Chapter 3). Over the years, Angle developed four appliances to treat patients without extractions. The objective behind these systems was to expand the arch form rather than using extractions to relieve crowding. The evolution of the Angle appliances is:

1) E-arch: the molar teeth were banded and every tooth was ligated to a heavy labial arch wire to deliver heavy interrupted forces. This appliance only allowed tipping of the teeth.
2) Pin and tube: more teeth in the arch were banded as well as the molars. A tube was soldered on to the bands to allow the heavy arch wire to pass through it. The pins had to be repositioned frequently to achieve the desired tooth movement.
3) Ribbon arch: the tubes on the band were modified with incorporation of a vertical slot and was termed bracket. A gold wire was engaged through the bracket slot and held in place with a pin to deliver light continuous forces. This appliance had great success yet presented with limited root control.
4) Edgewise: an evolution from the ribbon arch appliance is the edgewise system that provides much better crown and root control. After several experiments, the dimensions and orientation of the bracket slot altered. The edgewise system has a horizontal (90-degree) bracket slot. The width of the slot in the edgewise brackets are either 0.018 inch or 0.022 inch. A better control of the tooth movement is achieved as the wire closely fits in the bracket slot. The most popular brace systems known today are based on the edgewise appliance.

An Australian orthodontist Percy Raymond Begg launched the Begg technique on the fundamentals of the ribbon arch appliance. This technique was also designed for extraction cases. The edgewise technique focused on expanding the arch form without extractions and bodily movement of the teeth. However, the Begg technique involved a two-step tipping of the crown and uprighting the roots to achieve the desired tooth position with extractions to create the required space. The modifications made to the ribbon arch appliance to launch the Begg technique were:

- replacement of precious metal to stainless steel in the appliance.
- rotated the design of the bracket upside down.
- incorporated the use of auxiliary springs to adapt better root control.

Over the years, there has been several modifications made to the edgewise system yet all follow the same principle introduced by Angle. The non-extraction edgewise system was challenged by one of Angle's students, Charles H. Tweed. He introduced the use of edgewise appliances in combination with extractions and he formulated anchorage as a crucial aspect of a successful treatment. To enhance the efficiency of the edgewise appliance, the straight wire appliance was invented by Dr Lawrence Andrew and evolved by Dr Roth. This innovative technique incorporated torque and prescription angulation in the bracket slot to compensate for specific tooth anatomy. Integrating various angulations in different planes of space within the bracket design greatly reduced the need for several arch wire changes and bends in the final stages of treatment. However, bends in the wire for final detail is still critical to achieve the desired and ideal tooth position that varies in individuals. Other systems used a single bracket for every tooth and compensated for specific tooth movements using auxiliaries and repetitive bends in the arch wire. Owing to the prescriptions and variations in the design of the brackets, only one system can be used in an individual for optimum results. The bracket systems are differentiated on the basis of the slot width. The two main systems used are 0.018 inch and 0.022 inch with a depth variation between 0.025 inch and 0.032 inch.

### Self-Ligating Brackets

A revolution from the conventional brackets occurred with launching of self-ligating brackets in the early 1930s (Figure 5.2). Over several years, the design and mechanism of self-ligating brackets evolved and became more popular with the improved designs as treatment efficacy were enhanced. The self-ligating brackets have built-in gates or clips incorporated into the bracket to engage the arch wire without the need of modules. These brackets portray a significant improvement in oral hygiene due to less plaque accumulation without the presence of elastic modules holding the wire in place (Pellegrini, 2009).

Self-ligating brackets are differentiated in two categories based on their ligation mechanism (Brauchli et al., 2012) as:

1) Passive self-ligation: a gate built in the bracket to transform the open slot into a tube. This ligation mechanism offers a low friction system. Examples of passive self-ligating brackets include the Damon® System and SmartClip™ SL3 self-ligating appliance system.
2) Active self-ligation: a clip is incorporated in the bracket design that exerts pressure on the arch wire, thus enhances the effect by offering high control on tooth movement. The active clips provides enhanced rotational control and torque expression. Examples of self-ligating brackets are the Speed System™, In-Ovation® R and BioQuick®.

### Lingual Brackets

In the 1970s, lingual orthodontic appliances were introduced for better aesthetics. These appliances are used by many practitioners and require modified dexterity and specific lingual instruments. Initially, the desired outcomes were difficult to achieve because indirect vision made adjustments difficult. However, with development of software programs, customised brackets and wires for patients improved treatment outcomes dramatically (Figure 5.3). This innovation is used by many specialists, based on their training and experience.

### Components of Fixed Appliances

Precious metals and their alloys were first used in orthodontics before the Angle era. One of the most vital properties of these alloys were good corrosion resistance. However, poor tensile strength and flexibility were disadvantages. In 1919, Dr. F Hauptmeyer combined steel and chromium to introduce stainless steel with improved physical properties to replace gold in orthodontics. This combination has been widely used since the 1930s and are much more cost effective than gold. Arch wire can be manufactured from:

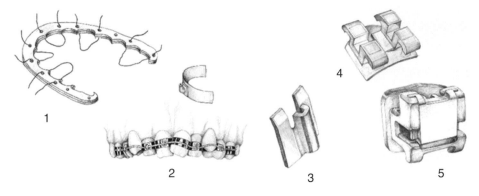

Figure 5.2 Evolution of brackets from the initial appliance introduce by Fauchard 1); evolving over several years to the ribbon arch 2); Begg 3); and the most commonly used bracket systems today, which are the conventional edgewise brackets 4); and the self-ligating brackets 5).

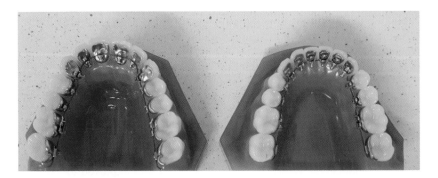

Figure 5.3 Lingual brackets.

- copper nickel titanium
- nickel titanium
- beta titanium
- chrome cobalt
- stainless steel
- gold alloy
- alpha titanium.

The physical properties vary depending on the shape, size and type of material. Fixed appliances contain active components and passive components. The active components of orthodontic appliances bring about the necessary movement. Examples of active components are arch wires, separator rings, elastics and coil springs. The passive components of fixed appliances deliver and transfer the force of active components; examples are brackets, bands, molar tubes and accessories such as modules.

### Active Components

### Arch Wires

The necessary physical properties of arch wire include stiffness, strength, flexibility, resilience, ductility, formability and biocompatibility. Stress is the ability to disperse the force load internally. There are three types of stress, which depends on the direction of force:

1) Tension (tensile strength).
2) Compression (compressive strength).
3) Shear stress.

Tensile stress results in elongation of the object, compressive stress condenses the object and shearing stress is the sliding of two objects against one another. Stress is associated with straining of the object. Strain is the distortion that occurs from stress and is categorised as elastic and plastic. Elastic strain reverses upon removal of the force and plastic strain is a permanent distortion to the object. The ratio of tensile stress to tensile stain is known as modulus of elasticity. This indicates the flexibility and stiffness of an object. The higher the modulus of elasticity, the higher the stiffness. Strength and stiffness are closely associated with range. Range is the elastic strain limitation prior to reaching a permanent internal deformation. The strength, stiffness and range of the arch wires are highly dependent on composition, shape, cross-section and size.

Resilience is another crucial physical property. The release and springback of energy that is absorbed by an object during stress is known as resilience. This generally happens before the object reaches its distortion limit. Ductility is the ability to undergo tensile forces and to withstanding plastic strain without breakage. Ductility decreases as the temperature increases. Malleability is undergoing plastic strain with compressive stress. Malleability increases with high temperatures. Formability is withstanding permanent distortions without material failure.

The ideal characteristics for an arch wire are low stiffness, high range, high strength and high formability. It may be difficult to gain all of these characteristics in one material, so various wires with different characteristics and materials are employed for specific purposes and to achieve the definite desired tooth movement.

The arch wire communicates the biomechanical forces through the brackets and tubes. The aim is to begin treatment with light continuous forces and gain effective tipping with round wires. The initial wire must have:

- sufficient flexibility
- resilience
- low stiffness
- high range
- freely move within the bracket slot.

An ideal arch wire for the initial stages of treatment must be biocompatible and should offer high resilience to spring back to its original shape upon force application. This allows sufficient alignment and precise tooth movement to be achieved with minimal distortions to the wire. The arch wires composed of nickel titanium alloy offer excellent elasticity and shape memory. Shape memory and thermoelasticity is the ability to regain initial form after deformation. The composition of the most commonly used arch wire is nickel, titanium, copper and chromium, and is available in round and rectangular cross sections. This wire is used as the initial wire in orthodontics due to its suitable physical properties.

The use of tightly fitted rectangular wires can create undesirable movements due to its effect on the root apex. However, better torque control is effectively achieved with arch wires that fully engage against the bracket slot. Stainless steel arch wires can be used from mid-treatment and for final finishing and detailing. Beta-titanium wires offer the most suitable physical properties for final detaining. The thickness and formability of these wires make them extremely effective. The detailing wires can be bent in the desired shape in the absence of material failure. As the diameter of the wire increases, the rigidity and stiffness also increases.

There have been several inventions in arch wire material and design to improve treatment efficacy, patient comfort, with the aim of minimising the need for frequent wire adjustments. Examples of some other arch wires include:

- Optiflex was a new invention to provide highly aesthetic clear arch wires. It can be used in cases of moderate crowding in the early stages of treatment. These tooth-coloured wires are composed of three optical fibres: silicon dioxide, which brings about tooth movement, silicon resin, which enhances moisture resistance and strength, and nylon, which adds strain resistance.
- Bioforce arch wire is another common shape memory alloy wire. It can undergo plastic deformation and return to its original shape. This thermodynamic arch wire contains gradient force across the arch wire, applying lower forces to the anterior section and increases towards the posterior and plateauing at the molars. It is an aesthetic wire and, with its force delivery, eliminates the need for frequent wire changes.
- Australian (Wilcock) arch wires are heat-treated stainless steel arches developed by Begg. Based on the resiliency of the wire, the Australian wire is categorised as round, regular, regular plus, special, special plus, premium, premium plus and supreme grades (Pelsue et al., 2009). The resiliency increases from regular to supreme. These wires are highly resistant to permanent deformation.

## Elastics

Synthetic elastomers and latex elastics are widely used in orthodontics. Latex elastics are composed of natural rubber and are used for intermaxillary traction. These elastics are also manufactured without latex for patients with latex allergy. The synthetic elastomers are composed of polyurethane rubber and are widely used for intramaxillary movement. Elastics vary in force and magnitude depending on several factors such as alveolar bone condition, patient cooperation and the movement required the choice of elastics vary. Different movements are achieved with several types of elastic patterns (discussed in Chapter 4).

## Springs

Nickel titanium coil springs provide continuous forces to open or maintain the space with open coils and closed coils, respectively.

## Passive Components

## Materials

Most brackets are composed of stainless steel containing chrome and nickel. There are plastic and ceramic brackets deigned for an aesthetic pleasing appearance. Plastic brackets are composed of polycarbonate and plexiglass. The problems associated with these types of brackets are poor physical properties and discolouration. The forces applied distort the bracket slot and the desired movements are not achieved, as the forces are not transmitted to the teeth appropriately. To resolve this issue, the plastic brackets were designed with stainless steel slots. Ceramic or fiberglass reinforced the material to improve the physical properties and colour stability. Ceramic brackets are made up of monocrystalline and polycrystalline. These brackets are highly fragile and have a high rate of breakage. Owing to the occlusal bearing in the posterior region and the risk of breakage, clear brackets are not manufactured for molars. The lowest friction is shown to be in ceramic reinforced composite brackets. Ceramic brackets can greatly damage enamel during the debonding process, due to the chemical retention mechanism of the resin in the orthodontic adhesives and the bracket base. To minimise enamel damage, the bonding mechanism is modified to a mechanical mode.

## Bonding

The brackets are designed with a mesh base of different types and patterns for better retention and bonding. There are various adhesives that can be used for orthodontic bonding with different modes of polymerisation (chemical, light or dual cured). Composite resin or resin reinforced glass ionomer cement are commonly used and the setting of the adhesives must be followed as recommended by the manufacturer. Brackets can be bonded to teeth with two different techniques, known as direct bonding or indirect bonding. Direct bonding is placement and positioning of each bracket directly on the enamel surface. Indirect bonding technique involves prepositioning the brackets on the cast models manually or on digital models using software programs. Once the ideal bracket positions are confirmed on the models by the orthodontist, plastic trays are fabricated over the brackets. Every specialist may have their own unique method of bonding. However, methods for bonding brackets using direct bonding (Figure 5.4) and indirect bonding (Figure 5.5) are summarised in Box 5.1.

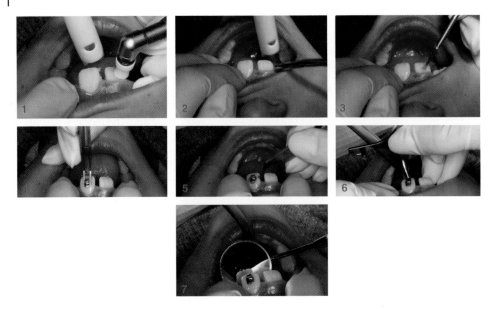

**Figure 5.4** Direct bonding. 1) Prophylaxis with pumice. 2) Wash and dry thoroughly. 3) Prepare all the teeth with etch and primer lollipop (it is recommended to microetch prior to this step to enhance bonding and minimise bonding failure). 4) Bracket directly placed on to the enamel surface. 5) Remove excess adhesive. 6) Check bracket placement using a height gauge. 7) Bracket placement is checked and the adhesive is set.

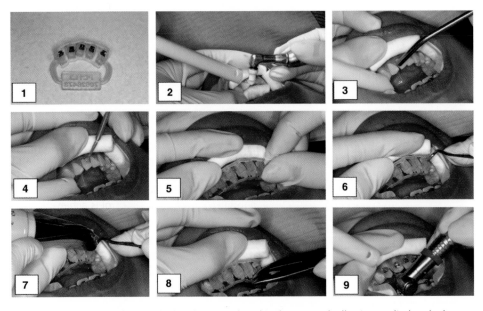

**Figure 5.5** Indirect bonding. 1) The brackets are placed in the tray and adhesive applied to the base. 2) The enamel surface is cleaned. 3) Pumice is washed and dried. 4) Etch and primer lollipop is applied over the tooth (after the enamel surface is micro etched). 5) The trays are secured over the teeth. 6) A firm pressure is applied with a pusher. 7) The adhesives are cured. 8) The trays are gently removed. 9) Excessive adhesive is polished surrounding the brackets.

---

**Box 5.1  Methods for Bonding Brackets in Direct and Indirect Bonding Methods**

### Direct Bonding

1) Prophylaxis of the enamel surface with pumice to remove pellicles, plaque and debris. A clean enamel surface maximises bond strength.
2) To enhance the bonding, the enamel surface is to be microetched with aluminium oxide. Ensure that the nozzle of the sand blaster is held away from the gingival margin to prevent soft tissue iatrogenic damage.
3) Wash and dry thoroughly to ensure that a clean enamel surface is achieved and that all surfaces are microetched (a shiny enamel surface is an indication that the enamel surface is not microetched).
4) A dry working field is extremely important to prevent bonding failures. Sufficient isolation is critical to prevent saliva contamination. Moisture control can be achieved with cotton rolls, dry tips, cheek and tongue retractors.
5) A self-etching primer lollipop is used to prepare the enamel surface prior to bonding. This eliminates the need for etch and applying bond in two steps. It allows the practitioner to etch, prime and bond in one simple step.
6) Brackets for each tooth are placed and positioned on the enamel using bracket tweezers. Excessive adhesive is removed surrounding the bracket.
7) The height of the bracket is checked with a height gauge.
8) Depending on the type adhesive used, the curing method differs and it may or may not require light activation. For an enhanced bonding strength, the appropriate polymerisation method for the adhesive must be followed and the patient must be advised accordingly. If the adhesive is chemically cured, the patient must be advised to avoid food or drink for about an hour to allow the setting of the adhesive to take place.

### Indirect Bonding

1) Impressions of teeth are taken and sent to laboratories or, if a software program is used, the teeth are scanned with a digital scanner and uploaded to the appropriate software.
2) The brackets are positioned on the plaster model or digitally positioned by the orthodontist on the software program.
3) Plastic trays are fabricated over the brackets.
4) The enamel preparation and moisture control do not differ from directing bonding.
5) Brackets are placed in the trays with adhesives on the base.
6) Once the enamel surface is ready for bonding and moisture control is achieved, the plastic trays are placed over the teeth.
7) Excessive adhesives are removed, polymerisation takes place and trays are gently removed.

---

### Positioning

Bracket placement and positioning must always be under the guidance and supervision of an orthodontist. The position of the bracket is extremely important in achieving the desired tooth movement. For the prescriptions and angulations incorporated in the bracket to work effectively, the bracket must be placed in the centre of the crown and along the long axis of the tooth. However, the type of bracket system used plays a role in bracket placement; for example, passive self-ligating bracket placement slightly differs from active self-ligating bracket placement to achieve harmony in the dental arches. The recommended bracket height is detailed in Table 5.1 but there are variations to this height, depending on the type and direction of tooth movement the specialist is trying to achieve. Variations in bracket placement is also commonly seen in patients with gingival hyperplasia, lingually or palatally displaced teeth and tooth size discrepancies. The vertical accuracy of the bracket placement is confirmed with the use of a height gauge (Figure 5.6). The gauges measure the height from the incisal and occlusal edges to the centre of the bracket slot.

Some suggestions for remembering bracket and molar tube placement are:

- Placement of the bracket too far gingivally will result in extrusion of the tooth. This is sometimes useful in bonding partially erupted teeth. However, in bonding molars this may not be ideal as the extrusion of the molars will lead to an anterior open bite as the posterior teeth will come into occlusion first.
- If the bracket is placed too far incisally, the tooth will be intruded.
- Distal placement of the bracket will cause the tooth to move mesially. Mesial placement of the bracket will move the tooth distally. This may aid in the correction of mild rotations to a degree.

Orthodontists will make modifications based on the anatomy and position of the tooth. In deep bite cases, the brackets are more incisally positioned in the anterior region and

Table 5.1 Average bracket placement.

| Teeth | Average Vertical Height (mm) |
| --- | --- |
| Upper: | |
| Central incisors | 5.0 |
| Lateral incisors | 4.5 |
| Canine | 5.0 |
| First premolar | 4.5 |
| Second premolar | 4.0 |
| First molar | 3.0 |
| Second molar | 2.0 |
| Lower: | |
| Central incisors | 4.0 |
| Lateral incisors | 4.0 |
| Canine | 4.5 |
| First premolar | 4.0 |
| Second premolar | 3.5 |
| First molar | 2.5 |
| Second molar | 2.5 |

more gingivally placed on the posterior region to open the bite with extrusion of the molars and intrusion of the anterior segment. In open bite cases, the brackets are positioned closer to the gingival margin in the anterior region to achieve a degree of extrusion (McLaughlin, 1999). Particular attention should be paid when bonding the second molars. If the molar tubes or brackets are positioned too far gingivally, an open bite will result from extrusion of the molars. This may be effective to mitigate deep bites but not ideal for every patient. It is important to check the position of the brackets at every visit to improve the efficiency of the treatment. If discrepancies in tooth position and bracket placements are noticed, the supervising orthodontist must immediately be notified to correct any inconsistencies by repositioning the brackets to achieve the desired movement.

Bite ramps are extremely useful on either the palatal surfaces of the central incisors or the occlusal surfaces of the molars to open the bite (Figure 5.7). This is to prevent maximum interdigitation of upper and lower arches to avoid bracket breakages or traumatic bites.

### Debonding the Brackets

Specific pliers are designed to make detachment of brackets possible with minimal enamel damage (Figure 5.8). Care must be given when debonding self-ligating brackets, as they can slide off the arch wire. Ceramic brackets must be removed from the base to

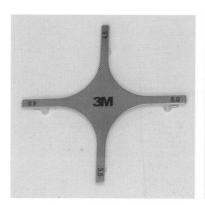
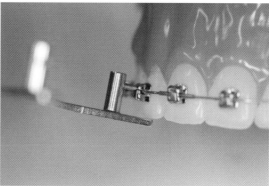

Figure 5.6 A height gauge is used to measure the height of the bracket from the incisal edge.

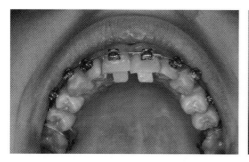
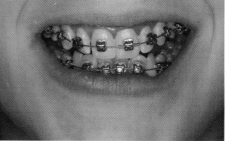

Figure 5.7 Bite ramps bonded to the palatal of the upper central incisors to prevent the upper teeth occluding on to the lower and causing bracket breakages.

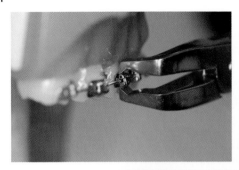
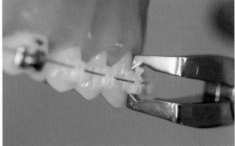
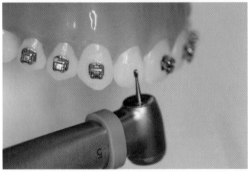

Figure 5.8 Debonding brackets. Clear brackets are removed from the base to prevent ceramic fracture.

prevent fracture. Carbide bur or polishing discs are used to remove the residual adhesive on the enamel. Always dry the enamel surface prior to removing the adhesive, to be able to distinguish enamel from the adhesive. In cases of ceramic fracture, diamond bur with high-speed handpieces are used to polish the ceramic remnants and the remaining adhesive is polished with a slow-speed polishing disc or bur to prevent enamel damage.

### Bands and Tubes

Molars are generally bonded with tubes or cemented with molar bands containing welded tubes. Bands are indicated in cases of gross restoration or teeth that are required to withstand heavy intermittent forces. Bands cover more surface area and thus can tolerate greater force. In some patients, it can be extremely difficult to maintain a dry working field in the molar region to prevent bonding failures, so banding the molars is a better option. Bonding tubes or molar brackets follow the same protocol as bonding other teeth, as discussed previously. Cementing bands, however, follows a different method. Space must be created between tight contacts of teeth to allow insertion of the bands interproximally. Doughnut-shaped elastics called separators are flossed between the teeth or positioned with a separating plier in tight contacts (Figure 5.9). This procedure is typically indicated two to seven days before band placement.

The most suitable size of molar band must be chosen to prevent complications after cementation. An ideal molar band should be seated firmly not tightly parallel with the molar marginal ridges. If the band is too large, gingival impingement can cause

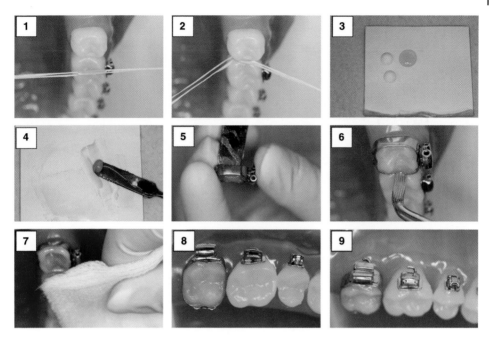

**Figure 5.9** Separators and banding. 1) and 2) Place separators between the teeth 2–7 days before the procedure and removed prior to banding. 3) Dispense the appropriate powder to liquid ratio. 4) Mix glass ionomer cement (GIC) to achieve a uniform material. 5) Load the band with GIC. 6) Adjust the band position with the band pusher. 7) Wipe the excess GIC. 8) and 9) Check the position of the band before setting the cement.

discomfort for the patient and the margins of the band will be positioned above the marginal ridges. The band can be dislodged soon after cementation if an incorrect size is selected. Once the ideal position and size of the band is identified, the working area is kept dry and the band is cemented with glass ionomer cement. The flush is removed and the position of the band is checked prior to setting the adhesive.

There are several types of adhesives used for bonding and banding fixed appliance components. Some may be chemically cured and others have a light-activated system. It is important to follow the correct procedures depending on the type of adhesive used to ensure the quality of the fit of the appliances. It is also important to know what type of adhesive is used so that patients can be advised accordingly. Chemically cured adhesive requires a certain amount of time to set, so patients must be advised to avoid food or drink for about one hour following treatment to avoid weak bonding. Light-activated systems eliminate this delay, as the adhesives set immediately once it is cured and food and drink do not impede the bonding strength.

### Accessories

Auxilliaries and accessories may be needed during orthodontic fixed appliance therapy to achieve the most desirable outcomes. There are several types of ligatures and auxiliaries available and some of the most commonly used are briefly explained in this section (Figure 5.10). An example is seen in Figure 5.11, using a figure eight steel ligature

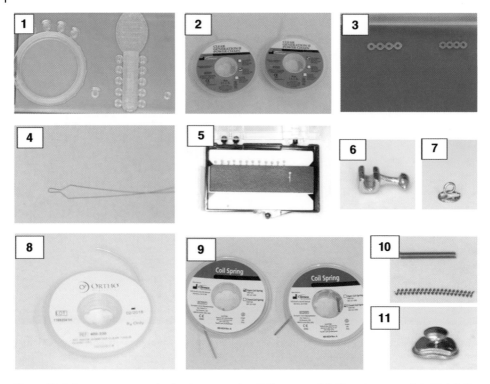

Figure 5.10 Some common orthodontic accessories. 1) Elastoguard (left), o-ring or module (right). 2) Open and closed power chains. 3) Close-up of open (left) and closed power chains (right). 4) Steel ligature. 5) Drop in pin. 6) Crimpable hooks. 7) Traction hook. 8) Elastic tubing or bumper sleeve. 9) Spring coil. 10) Close-up of closed spring coil (top) and open spring coil (bottom). 11) button.

tie to hold the teeth together prior to insertion of the arch wire. Every specialist will have their own unique style of work and these accessories can be incorporated as part of fixed appliance therapy in several ways, which greatly varies among specialists. Some of the basic functions of certain auxiliaries are outlined in Table 5.2.

## Oral Hygiene and Maintenance

Providing oral hygiene and care is one of the primary roles of oral health therapists, dental hygienists and dental therapists (Figure 5.12). Extensive knowledge in this area and providing patients with sufficient valuable information can greatly minimise complications associated with poor oral hygiene. Oral hygiene education and diet advice can be reviewed at every appointment, particularly if signs of gingivitis and visible plaque accumulation around the appliances are evident. It is extremely effective to demonstrate the oral hygiene advice given and allowing patients to practise to help them gain a better understanding once an appliance is fitted or bonded (Box 5.2).

A poor oral hygiene regimen results in decalcification and gingivitis, and can lead to periodontitis. Diet plays a critical role in maintaining a healthy oral health environment. Poor diet not only results in high risk of caries but can also cause significant damage to the appliance. Patients undergoing orthodontic therapy must avoid hard and sticky food

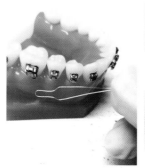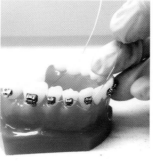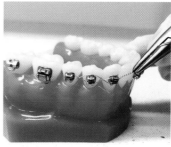

Figure 5.11  A long steel ligature tie in a figure of eight around the brackets.

Table 5.2  Some basic functions of auxiliaries and accessories.

| Auxilliary | Description |
|---|---|
| Modules | Elastomers or steel ligature ties are used to ligate and engage the wire with the bracket, increasing friction and to initiate tooth movement. Elastoguard as shown on the left in Figure 5.10 (1) is used to protect the bracket from the occlusion and to prevent breakage by guarding the bracket (application is shown in Figure 5.7). |
| Power chain | Used to engage the wire against the bracket and used for grouping teeth (holding the teeth together and close spaces). There are two types of power chains with different force strength:<br>• closed (higher tension)<br>• open (lower tension). |
| Steel ligature tie | Long steel ligature ties can be tied around the brackets in a figure of eight. Short steel ligature ties can aid in ligating the arch wire to the bracket. |
| Drop-in pin | Placed in the auxiliary bracket slot for elastic wear. There are numerous designs to these pins or hooks depending on the type of bracket system used. |
| Crimpable hooks | Placed on the arch wire prior to surgery by the specialist for ligation during the surgery. Also can be added to arch wire for elastic wear. |
| Bondable traction hook with round eyelet | Typically bonded on exposed teeth and are ligated in various ways to traction the tooth in to alignment. |
| Elastic tube | Known as arch wire sleeve/tubing or bumper sleeve to protect the lip from the wire in long spans and maintain spaces in areas of missing teeth. |
| Spring coil | An open coil is used to create spaces once activated. A closed coil is used to maintain spaces. |
| Closed coil | Measured exactly to the space that needs to be maintained. |
| Open coil | Can be activated via the addition of a small closed coil or cutting the open coil about half a bracket width longer than the space required. There numerous ways in which an open coil can be activated and each specialist can have their own unique method. |
| Button | Can be bonded onto various tooth surfaces for elastic wear or power chains. It can be bonded palatal, lingual or buccal depending on the need. |

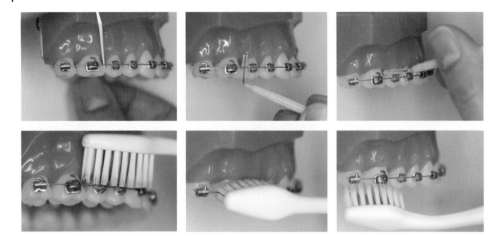

Figure 5.12 Orthodontic oral hygiene.

---

**Box 5.2  Patient Oral Hygiene Advice**

**Fixed appliances**

- Brush three times a day: in the morning after breakfast, after lunch and after dinner.
- Floss can be used to clean between the teeth using a floss threader for better guidance of the floss under the wire; alternatively, super floss can be used.
- Interdental brushes must be used interproximally to clean the lateral surfaces of the brackets and teeth, as the wire prevents the toothbrush bristles from reaching those areas.
- The toothbrush must be held at a 45-degree angle to reach and clean the gingival margin, top surfaces of the brackets and under the brackets.
- Fluoridated toothpaste should be used to help to remineralise early decalcification and to help protect the enamel.
- Mouthwash can be used after meals if necessary; however, the plaque must be physically removed using the correct techniques. Mouthwash should not replace brushing.
- Electric toothbrushes have been shown to be more effective and are highly recommended for children, who have a lower dexterity.

**Removable appliances**

- The patient must always wear the appliances as instructed by the clinician.
- All appliances should be cleaned with cold water and a toothbrush.
- A minimal amount of toothpaste must be used, as it can be too abrasive on the appliances.
- Avoid denture cleaning products, as these can be too abrasive for the acrylic materials used for the appliances.
- Protect appliances in cases when they are not being worn.

in particular, to prevent breakage and damage to the appliance. A soft food diet for at least one week is recommended to aid in reducing initial discomfort. The patient must be made aware that treatment time can be affected with constant breakage and damage to the appliance, so, attention must be paid to avoiding foods that can harm braces or other fixed appliances.

Patient motivation is key for sufficient oral hygiene and good diet. Therefore, at every visit, the clinician is responsible for checking the fit of the appliances, oral health and hygiene of the patient and ensuring that the patient is not in any discomfort caused by ill-fitting appliances. Extra time should be dedicated to help to motivate the patient. Written instructions on diet, oral hygiene and common emergencies must always be issued. In the initial stages of orthodontic treatment, patients and their families are particularly apprehensive regarding emergencies and how to handle them. They need to be provided with information and guidance on how to manage an emergency situation until they get in contact with their orthodontic clinic. Patients must be notified of what situations are considered as orthodontic emergencies. It is not always a trauma to the head and neck that can result in emergencies. Broken bands, brackets and ill-fitting appliances causing ulceration and discomfort are all considered orthodontic emergencies. For example, eating sticky food can result in broken brackets or broken arch wires and the patient must know not to ignore this matter until their next regular check-up. They should know how to use the orthodontic wax to alleviate any sharpness and secure the wire or bracket in place until treatment is pursued as soon as possible.

As clinicians, it is vital to gain sufficient information on the cause of the emergencies to eliminate unwanted situations as much as possible. Repeated broken appliances play a significant role in delayed orthodontic treatment.

## Orthodontic Instruments

Special instruments are manufactured for orthodontic purposes. The basic general instruments, such as a dental mirror, explorer and probe, are not discussed here. The aim of this section is to identify some of the widely used orthodontic instruments. Many of the pliers and orthodontic instruments have modified designs dedicated to lingual braces to allow better access and placement of brackets, arch wires and ligatures lingually. Clinicians must have sufficient knowledge of orthodontic instrumentation to prevent misuse and damage. Orthodontic pliers are designed with a round tip for patient safety, as hard metal is used for manufacturing the tip of the instruments. Stainless steel and tungsten carbide are the two most common materials used for the tips of cutting instruments. Each material has advantages and disadvantages. Tungsten carbide can have a higher durability, provide greater grip, sharp cutting edge but it can be very brittle. One of the greater advantages of stainless steel is corrosion resistance.

### Adjustment Instruments

Some common adjustment instruments include:

- Weingart pliers: used to hold arch wires and guide them through brackets (no. 1, Figure 5.13).

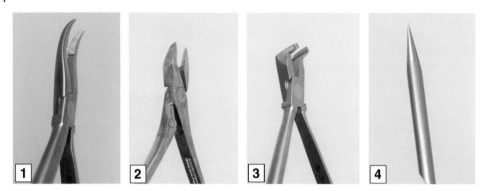

Figure 5.13 Some common wire adjustment instruments: 1) Weingart pliers. 2) Ligature cutter. 3) Distal end cutter. 4) Example of a self-ligating opening tool.

- Ligature cutter: used to cut wires and ligatures (no. 2, Figure 5.13).
- Distal end cutter: used to trim the distal ends of the arch wires (no. 3, Figure 5.13). These cutters are designed with magnetic tips to enhance safety and may be used both intraorally and extraorally.
- Self-ligating opening tool: self-ligating brackets require specific tools to open the gates or clips on the brackets (no. 4, Figure 5.13). Each bracket system has a different design to the opening tool that fits the gates or clips.
- Howe pliers: aid in holding arch wires. Howe pliers are designed as straight or curved. The curved version is best used for posterior regions.

### Bracket Placement Instruments

Bracket tweezers are also known as a bracket holders or placers. They are used to hold the brackets for direct bonding (no. 1, Figure 5.14). Some bracket tweezers are designed with a flat end on the handle that can allow better positioning of the bracket once

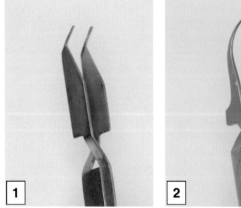
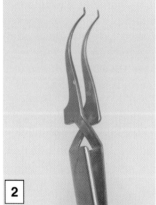
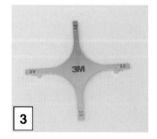

Figure 5.14 Some common bracket placement instruments: 1) Anterior bracket tweezers. 2) Posterior bracket tweezers; the curvature in the tip allows better access posteriorly. 3) Height gauge.

inserted in the slot. Bracket tweezers with a curvature on the tip are used for posterior bonding (no. 2, Figure 5.14).

A height gauge is used to measure the height of the bracket from the incisal edge (no. 3, Figure 5.14). The flat edge rests on the incisal edges and the pointed tip rests in the bracket slot.

### Bracket Removing Instruments

There are two different types of debonding pliers used for removing metal and clear brackets. Angled pliers are designed for retraction of the cheek and better access to the posterior region (no. 1, Figure 5.15). Straight pliers are designed for anterior teeth (no. 2, Figure 5.15). Ceramic brackets must be removed from the base, so there are pliers with a unique design to make this possible without fracturing the brackets (no. 3, Figure 5.15).

### Banding Instruments

- Band-removing pliers: anterior and posterior band-removing pliers are designed to detach the bands (no. 1, Figure 5.16). The plastic tip of the plier rests on the occlusal surface of the tooth as the metal tip rests on the gingival border of the band. The band is removed once pressures is exerted on the handles and pulled towards the occlusal or lingual.
- Band pusher: used to cement and seat bands firmly around the tooth (no. 2, Figure 5.16). Designed with a serrated tip and a cylindrical handle.
- Band seater: the serrated tip, which comes in various shapes (triangular, rectangular or circular), allows better placement of bands (no. 3, Figure 5.16). It is seated inter-proximally on the edge of the band and the patient bites on the stick handle. The firm pressure from the bite allows the band to be seated correctly around the tooth. This instruments is particularly useful in seating bands subgingivally.

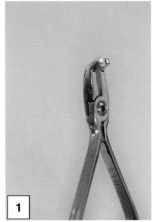 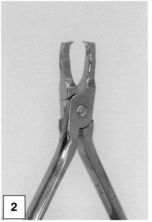 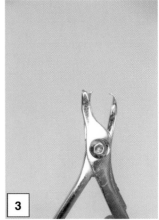

Figure 5.15 Bracket-removing pliers: 1) Posterior debonding pliers. 2) Anterior debonding pliers. 3) Debonding pliers for ceramic brackets.

### Wire-Forming Pliers

- Adams pliers: aid in forming the clasps and adjusting plates (no. 1, Figure 5.17).
- Torque pliers: create bends in the wire to achieve the desired torque once the wire is engaged with the bracket (no. 2, Figure 5.17).
- Tweed: designed for bending and loop-forming; aids in placing bends in the wire for detailing (no. 3, Figure 5.17).
- Bird-beak pliers: used for preparing and forming the arch wire. Commonly used for forming detailing wires (no. 4, Figure 5.17).
- Jaraback pliers: used for loops, bending and forming arch wires.
- Ribbon-arch pliers: loop-forming pliers.
- V-bending pliers: forms a V-shaped loop in steel and titanium arch wires.
- Mathieu needle-holding pliers: used for ligation and holding ligatures (no. 1, Figure 5.18).
- Ligature adjustor and tucker: aids in holding the arch wires and ligatures in place (no. 2, Figure 5.18). It is extremely useful for bending and pushing the arch wires for better placement in the bracket slots.
- Mosquito forceps: used for holding ligatures (no. 3, Figure 5.18). Very similar to Mathieu's pliers.

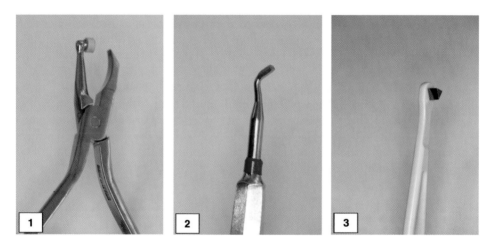

Figure 5.16  Banding instruments: 1) Band remover. 2) Band pusher. 3) Band seater/band biter.

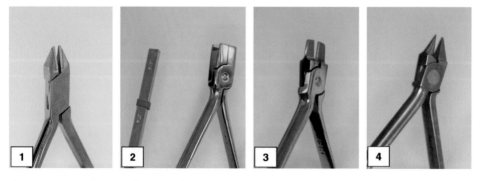

Figure 5.17  Wire-forming pliers: 1) Adams pliers. 2) Torque pliers. 3)Tweed. 4) Bird-beak plier.

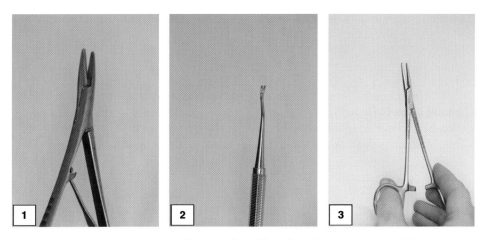

Figure 5.18  Other instruments: 1) Mathieu needle-holding pliers. 2) Ligature tucker. 3) Mosquito forceps.

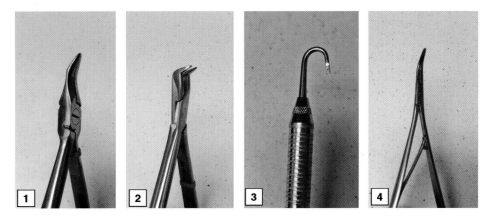

Figure 5.19  1) Lingual weingart pliers. 2) Lingual cutter (the curve in the tip makes this cutter resemble a distal end cutter. 3) Lingual ligature tucker. 4) Lingual mosquito forceps.

### Lingual Instruments

Lingual instruments have a 45-degree bend at the tip to facilitate placement of wires and ligatures (Figure 5.19).

## References

Brauchli, L. M., Steineck, M., Wichelhaus, W. Active and passive self-ligation: a myth? *Angle Orthod*, 2012; 82(4): 663–669.

McLaughlin, R. P., Bennett, J. C., Trevisi, H. Practical techniques for achieving improved accuracy in bracket positioning. *Orthod Perspect*, 1999; 6(1): 21–24.

Pellegrini, P., Sauerwein, R., Finlayson, T. Plaque retention by self-ligating vs elastomeric orthodontic brackets: Quantitative comparison of oral bacteria and detection with adenosine triphosphate-driven bioluminescence. *Am J Orthod Dentofacial Orthop*, 2009; 135(4): 426.e1–9.

Pelsue, B. M., Zinelis, S., Bradley, T. G., et al. Structure, composition, and mechanical properties of Australian orthodontic wires. *Angle Orthod*, 2009; 79(1): 97–101

## Further Reading

Ajlouni, R., Bishara, S. E., Oonsombat, C., et al. Evaluation of modifying the bonding protocol of a new acid-etch primer on the shear bond strength of orthodontic brackets. *Angle Orthod*, 2004; 74(3): 410–413.

Bishara, S. E. *Textbook of Orthodontics*. Philadelphia, PA: W.B. Saunders; 2001.

Foster, T. D. *A Textbook of Orthodontics*. 3rd ed. Oxford: Blackwell Scientific; 1990.

Mitchell, L. *An Introduction to Orthodontics*. 3rd ed. Oxford: Oxford University Press; 2007.

## Self-Evaluation

1 Who is known as the father of orthodontics?
   A Edward Hartley Angle.
   B Pierre Fauchard.
   C Charles H. Tweed.
   D Percy Raymond Begg.

2 From what materials can fixed appliances be manufactured?
   A Nickel titanium.
   B Chromium cobalt.
   C Gold alloy.
   D All of the above (a–c).

3 Which of the following materials offer the highest elasticity and memory shape?
   A Stainless steel.
   B Chromium cobalt.
   C Nickel titanium.
   D Beta titanium.

4 Which type of wire offers the highest torque control?
   A Rectangular cross-section.
   B Round cross-section.
   C a and b.
   D Triangular cross-section.

5 By which mechanics can bracket adhesives bond to enamel?
   A Chemical bonding.
   B Micromechanical bonding.
   C a and b.
   D None of the above.

6   What is the difference between a closed-coil spring and an open-coil spring?
    **A**  Closed-coil spring create spaces for tooth movement.
    **B**  Active open-coil springs create spaces for eruptions only.
    **C**  Closed-coil springs close extraction spaces.
    **D**  Closed-coil springs maintain spaces in the arch, while active open-coil springs create spaces.

7   Which type of brackets present with reduced plaque retention?
    **A**  Self-ligating brackets.
    **B**  Conventional brackets.
    **C**  Begg brackets.
    **D**  Ribbon arch.

8   Which of the following are NOT considered an active component of fixed appliances?
    **A**  Arch wires.
    **B**  Elastics.
    **C**  Springs.
    **D**  Brackets.

9   What instrument is commonly used to hold and guide arch wires through the bracket slots?
    **A**  Ligature director.
    **B**  Weingart pliers.
    **C**  Mathieu pliers.
    **D**  Bracket tweezers.

10  What is considered the ideal bracket position?
    **A**  Closer to the incisal edge.
    **B**  Closer to the gingival margin.
    **C**  On the midline of the tooth.
    **D**  Closer to the side of rotation.

# 6

# Treatment for Class I Malocclusion

Chapters 6–11 outline some of the treatment objectives and principles of various malocclusions and skeletal discrepancies. Cases are presented throughout the chapters to help oral health therapists and dental hygienists to gain a better understanding of some of the possible treatments carried out by orthodontists. The mechanics and details of treatment modalities are not discussed in depth, as these are beyond the scope of this textbook.

   The objective of treating class I malocclusion is correction of the dental discrepancies, as patients typically present with a favourable soft tissue environment and harmonious skeletal structures, with an exception for bimaxillary cases. Some of the dental concerns seen in class I malocclusion are discussed in this chapter, although these are not confined to class I and are common in other malocclusions. Examples of these dental concerns include spacing, crowding, ectopic teeth, impacted teeth, cross bites and open bites.

## Spacing and Crowding

The decision on how to close excessive spaces or relief crowding depends on some of the following factors:

- the skeletal profile of the patient
- the type of malocclusion
- the degree of crowding
- the inclination of the teeth
- the space available
- the space needed for correction of the malocclusion.

### Spacing

Spacing can occur because of congenitally missing teeth, premature tooth loss, microdontia, fraenal attachment to the incisive papilla or supernumeraries. The cause of spacing must be eliminated if possible; for example, frenectomy is indicated if a median diastema is due to a large labial fraenum. Typically, a periapical radiograph is also necessary in cases with a median diastema to check for presence of supernumeraries.

*Orthodontics for Dental Hygienists and Dental Therapists*, First Edition. Tina Raked.
© 2018 John Wiley & Sons Ltd. Published 2018 by John Wiley & Sons Ltd.
Companion website: www.wiley.com/go/raked/orthodontics_dental_hygienists

**Primary Dentition**

Excessive spaces in the primary dentition are monitored and active treatment is not indicated.

**Mixed Dentition**

Spacing can be monitored in mild cases, depending on the age of the patient, aetiology and degree of spacing. Mild divergence and increased spacing between the upper incisors between the ages of 7 and 12 years can be considered normal (the 'ugly duckling' stage) and is corrected upon eruption of the upper canines.

During the mixed dentition stage, the premature loss of posterior teeth (particularly the primary second molars) can be an issue, as there is a risk of a mesial drift of the permanent first molars. In these cases, a space maintainer is necessary to preserve the space for the eruption of the permanent successors. Examples of space maintainers include the Nance holding appliance (Figure 6.1A) and the lower lingual holding arch (Figure 6.1B) and the transpalatal arch (Figure 6.1C). This also aims at preventing a midline shift in early loss of deciduous canines.

**Permanent Dentition**

Excessive spaces can be treated with a series of clear aligners if there is a favourable soft-tissue environment in the absence of severe skeletal discrepancies. Space closure is also easily achieved with fixed appliances. If the space is due to tooth loss, an option would be creating sufficient space with fixed appliances for an implant or bridge,

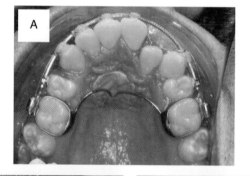

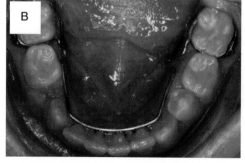
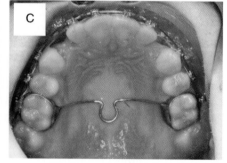

Figure 6.1 A) Nance B) LLHA (Lower Lingual Holding Arch C) TPA (Transpalatal Arch).

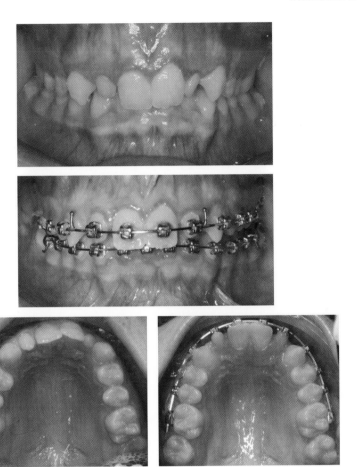

Figure 6.2 Comparing the initial and mid-treatment photographs, it is evident that space is gained mesial and distal to the peg lateral incisors to allow sufficient space for restorative composite resin build-up. *Source*: Case by Dr Shimanto K. Purkayastha.

depending on the periodontal health status. A combination of orthodontic and restorative treatment provides optimum results in cases of microdontia and peg laterals (Figures 6.2 and 6.3).

### Crowding

A size discrepancy between the dental arches and teeth leads to crowding. The space needed for the correction of crowding can be achieved in several ways, such as arch expander appliances or extraction for large spaces and active open-coil spring for gaining minor spaces.

### Primary Dentition

Crowding at this early stage is due to a lack of primate spaces (see Chapter 3) and is an indication that crowding will occur in the permanent dentition. Regular check-ups are therefore critical and the eruption of the permanent teeth must be monitored closely.

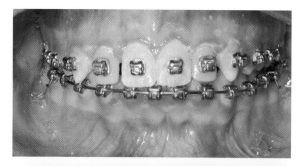

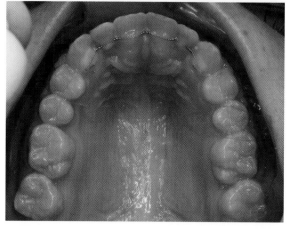

**Figure 6.3** Composite resin build-up of peg lateral incisors. Final detailing and space closures were achieved. Fixed lingual retainers are used for retention post treatment to enhance the stability.

### Mixed Dentition

In mild to moderate crowding resulting in ectopic eruption or impaction of permanent teeth, phase I treatment aids in creating space in several ways. In mild cases, the incisors are grouped by partial fixed-appliance therapy (known as 2 × 4; see Chapter 3). Once sufficient space is created, a fixed lingual retainer is placed on the palatal of the incisors to prevent relapse after the fixed appliances are removed. The eruption of the permanent dentition is monitored and space maintainers are bonded to preserve the space. The aim of this early intervention is to prevent severe crowding in the permanent dentition, to prevent ectopic eruptions and to eliminate the need for extraction of permanent teeth for gaining space once growth is ceased.

Before the growth spurt occurs, an expander plate, such as a the rapid maxillary expander, or a slow maxillary expander (quad helix) is used to create spaces in narrow arches. This type of treatment can be used in combination with partial braces to align the erupted teeth once sufficient space has been gained with the use of an expander.

### Permanent Dentition

Mild to moderate crowding in the absence of skeletal discrepancies can be treated with a series of aligners. A tipping movement of only one or two teeth can be achieved with the use of a removable appliance. High patient compliance is necessary for optimum results with removable appliances.

Beyond the growth spurt and in cases of severe crowding, extractions are indicated. The decision for extraction is always made by an orthodontist. In adults, the need for space maintainers is highly dependent on the degree of anchorage needed. Extractions are therefore always carefully planned with sufficient anchorage in adults.

## Case Study

An example of treating crowding using fixed appliance therapy is seen in the case presented in Figures 6.4 and 6.5. The patient presented with:

- brachyfacial
- convex profile
- facial symmetry
- competent lips
- an anterior traumatic deep bite
- overretained upper right deciduous canine.

Further findings of significance indicated that the roots of the upper incisor teeth appear long and slender and there appeared to be some root curvature in the apical thirds of the central incisors. The treatment objectives of the patient and the specialist were to:

- improve the facial profile
- improve the soft-tissue lip pattern
- improve the skeletal base relationship
- correct overjet and overbite
- develop the upper arch form
- relieve crowding
- align and level the dental arches
- coordinate the dental arch forms
- align and coordinate the centre lines
- establish a class I molar relationship
- establish a class I canine relationship
- reduce or eliminate any temporomandibular joint pain and/or discomfort
- reduce or eliminate any psychosocial issues re: teeth and smile
- allow normal eruption of permanent teeth
- reduce the need for (or severity of) phase II orthodontic treatment
- produce stable treatment results.

The patient was referred for extraction of the overretained primary upper right canine prior to orthodontic treatment. Upper and lower fixed appliances using a self-ligating 0.022-inch preadjusted edgewise prescription with selective torques were fitted. Once a degree of alignment was achieved, fixed class II orthopaedic appliances (Forsus™) were fitted to address the skeletal class II (discussed in Chapter 7). Upon completion of the treatment, fixed lingual retainers in the upper and lower arches with a removable maxillary retainer for the upper arch were planned for retention. The patient was kept on a recall system for monitoring of the eruption of the third permanent molars.

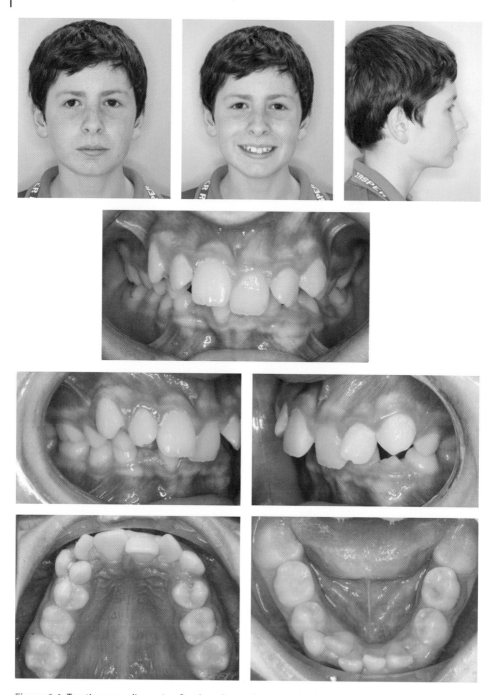

Figure 6.4 Treating crowding using fixed appliance therapy; initial records. *Source*: Case by Dr Shimanto K. Purkayastha.

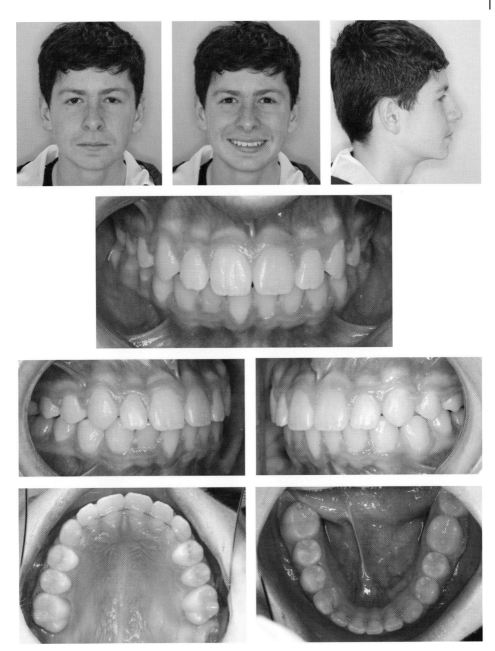

Figure 6.5 Treating crowding using fixed appliance therapy; final records. *Source*: Case by Dr Shimanto K. Purkayastha.

## Ectopic and Impacted Canines

Ectopic eruption is the term given to a tooth that erupts in a position other than its norm. Canines are one of the most commonly ectopic teeth. The aetiology of canine displacement is not fully understood. Ectopic canines can be associated with crowding, overretained primary canines, hereditary factors, displacement of the crypt, a short-rooted upper lateral incisor or the absence of the upper lateral incisor (Mitchell, 2001). Clinically, the canines should be palpable distal to the lateral incisors as a buccal bulge in the gingiva, at around the age of 9 years and above. Radiographic investigations, such as orthopantograms, periapicals, occlusal radiographs, lateral cephalometrics or computed tomography (CT), may be indicated if canines are not palpable in the labial sulcus or asymmetrical eruptions are detected. In case of an ectopic or impacted canine, the position of the crown, the root apex and its effect on the surrounding dentition must be examined carefully using radiographs. It is vital to determine whether the canine is palatally or buccally impacted. The position of the tooth is better examined on three-dimensional CT.

In severe cases, the canine is surgically exposed and space is created with fixed appliances to traction the canine into the ideal position. In some cases, the canine is transposed. Transposition is the change of position of two teeth. Depending on the clinical findings of the specialist, the position of the canine will be interchanged with an adjacent tooth. This is commonly seen in cases where the ectopic tooth has caused significant damage to the root of the adjacent tooth. If the damaged tooth has a poor prognosis, it will be replaced with the ectopic tooth in that area. This type of treatment will involve cosmetic restoration to contour the shape of the tooth in the occlusion.

### Case Study

An example of exposure and alignment of an impacted canine is presented in Figures 6.6, 6.7 and 6.8. The patient presented with:

- crowding of the upper and lower anterior teeth
- 100% overbite
- asymmetric bite
- retruded upper and lower anterior segments
- palatal impaction of the upper left canine
- microdontic upper lateral incisors; the upper right incisor was markedly peg shaped
- the incisors presented with short and thin roots radiographically.

The treatment plan was:

- Placement of a transpalatal holding arch with incorporation of a mini-screw to supplement anchorage.
- Exposure of the impacted upper left canine, bonded with a nickel–titanium spring upon exposure and attached to the transpalatal arch to extrude the tooth and move it posteriorly away from the roots of the maxillary incisors. The reason for this was that if fixed appliances were to be placed on the maxillary incisors, the crown of these teeth (given how retroclined they were) would flare forward and the roots would move palatally and contact the crown of the upper left impacted canine. Given the increased risk for root resorption due to the short thin roots, the orthodontist wanted to avoid this situation as much as possible.
- Placement of the fixed appliances in the upper arch once the impacted canine was extruded palatally.

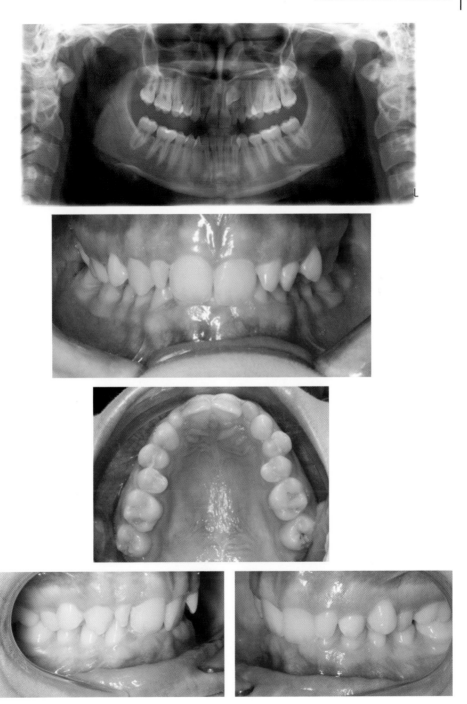

Figure 6.6 Exposure and alignment of an impacted canine; initial records. *Source*: Case by Dr Shimanto K. Purkayastha.

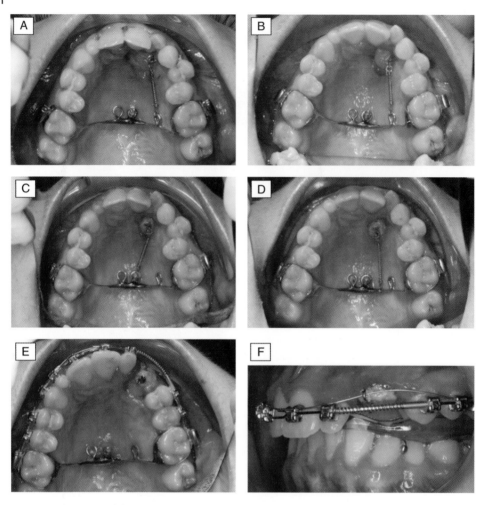

**Figure 6.7** Exposure of the impacted canine: A) Upon exposure. B) one month post-exposure. C) Three months post-exposure. D) Five months post-exposure. E) Two years post-exposure. F) Two years post-exposure, issued with a lower bite plane to traction the canine into the arch.

- Once the upper left canine was moved labially, lower fixed appliances were fitted.
- Composite enlargement of the lateral incisors.
- Retention involving a fixed lingual retainer in both arches.

### Risks of Impaction

The risks and problems associated with impacted teeth include ankylosis of the tooth as it becomes fused to the bone. The traction of an ankylosed tooth will not be possible without additional surgical procedures. In some cases, extraction of the impacted tooth and replacement with implants or bridges may be required. The impacted tooth or the adjacent teeth can lose vitality and may need subsequent treatment such as root canal therapy.

Periodontal complications associated with the impacted tooth may indicate a need for bone grafting to make further treatment possible. Impacted teeth can damage the roots of the adjacent teeth if left untreated.

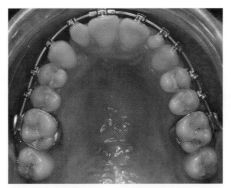

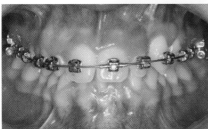
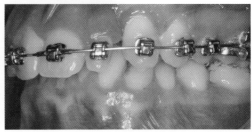

**Figure 6.8** Extraction of the overretained deciduous canine took place and the left canine was aligned in the arch. The next stages of the treatment involved creating space for the build-up of the upper lateral incisors and bonding lower arch braces to bring the dental arches in harmony (courtesy of Dr Shimanto K. Purkayastha).

## Cross Bite

Cross bite is a transverse discrepancy of the dental arches. It may occur unilaterally, bilaterally, posteriorly or anteriorly. In posterior cross bites, the buccal cusps of the posterior lower teeth occlude on the buccal cusps of the upper posterior teeth. If the entire segment is positioned lingually or buccally in relation to the opposing arch, it is termed 'scissor bite' (also known as a lingual cross bite). A common clinical finding of a unilateral cross bite is displacement of the mandible, with lateral shifts upon closure to get maximum interdigitation. If left untreated, this may lead to temporomandibular joint disorders. Common causes of cross bites include:

- displacement of the permanent tooth bud due to trauma
- inconsistency in the arch length as a result of growth deficiencies in the jaws
- lack of space due to overretained deciduous teeth or supernumeraries
- cleft palate.

### Posterior Cross Bite

Transverse or anteroposterior discrepancies results in posterior cross bites. A rapid maxillary expander or a slow maxillary expander such as a quad helix is used if the maxilla is too narrow. Expanders separate sutures and widen the arch once it is activated. This treatment is most suitable during active growth. Studies show that early use of expanders in the primary dentition is not advisable as it can cause distortion to the nasal bony structure as the two bony plates in the palate are separated. This occurs because of the close proximity of the nasal floor and the bony palates.

Depending on the severity of the malocclusion, fixed appliances are used in combination with an expander for further correction and alignment of the occlusion. There are two types of rapid maxillary expanders: banded and bonded (Figures 6.9–6.11). The expansion plate is activated to separate the palatal suture. The rate and amount of expansion is calculated and decided by the orthodontist and varies for every patient, depending on the degree of space required for correction of the malocclusion. The plate is activated for a certain period of time but left in place passively for around six months to allow sufficient bone growth and infill of the suture. Early removal of the plate leads to relapse due to soft tissue pressure.

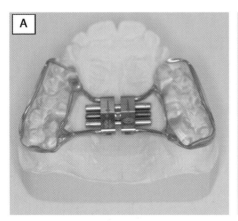 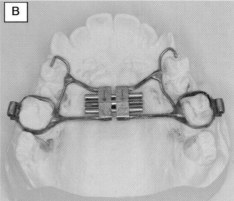

Figure 6.9 A rapid maxillary expander (RME) with hex screw: A) Bonded RME; the acrylic-based RME covers more teeth and offers higher anchorage. This expander is typically used in open bite cases to prevent further extrusion of the molars and mitigate the open bite effect. B) Banded RME; the expander is designed with bands on the upper first molars and first premolar. Some expanders are designed with rests on the premolars or primary first molars instead of bands as shown. Upon expansion, the molars are extruded to a degree.

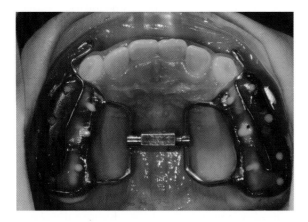

Figure 6.10 Bonded rapid maxillary expander with a superscrew.

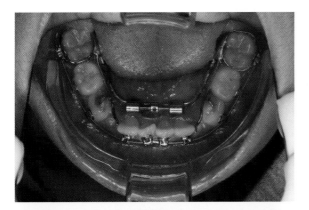

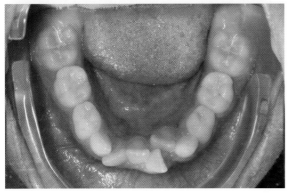

Figure 6.11 Expanders designed for the lower arch. *Source*: Case by Dr Shimanto K. Purkayastha.

Some indications for maxillary expansion are bilateral constricted maxilla, deficient maxilla, high narrow palate and maxillary collapse seen in cleft palate. Maxillary expansion can be achieved in two ways:

1) Rapid: requires patient control and higher magnitude of force; widening the palatal suture improves airway flow.
2) Slow: does not require patient control, takes a prolonged period of time and has low force.

### Anterior Cross bite

One of the most effective ways to correct anterior cross bite is with the use of fixed appliances and a removable lower bite plane. The objective of the treatment is to retrocline the lower teeth in a cross bite as the upper teeth are proclined. However, other treatment options may be undertaken for individual variations such as age, facial growth pattern and the skeletal discrepancy presented by the patient.

### Permanent Dentition

Posterior cross bites are most effectively treated in adults with the use of cross elastics during fixed appliance therapy (see Chapter 4 for elastic wear). Anterior cross bites can effectively be treated in adults with fixed appliances and a bite plane. However, if the cross bit is accompanied by severe skeletal discrepancies, a surgical approach may be indicated.

## Open Bite

Open bite refers to the failure of vertical overlap between the upper and lower jaws. The defect may be anterior or posterior. Common characteristics of an open bite include:

- a narrow maxillary arch
- mandibular deficiency
- posterior cross bite
- overeruption of incisors
- incompetent lips
- sigmatism (lisping)
- increased lower facial height.

Aetiological factors for this type of malocclusion can be digit sucking, lip or tongue habits, airway obstruction and skeletal growth abnormalities (Ngan, 1997). Studies suggest that airway obstruction and mouth breathing are not significant in the aetiology of an anterior open bite. However, some cases have been found associating airway obstruction to increased lower facial heights.

### Primary Dentition

The eruption of the adult teeth must be monitored closely and if the open bite is due to digit sucking, the habit must be ceased using various techniques to prevent the open bite being transmitted to the permanent dentition as well.

### Mixed Dentition

In mild cases with favourable soft tissue and growth, the patient can be treated with orthodontic appliances. Some orthodontists might plan a treatment involving intrusion of the molars rather than extrusion of the incisors, for a better prognosis and treatment stability. This can be achieved with the use of high-pull headgear. The maxillary growth is restrained by intrusive forces by wearing the appliance for 14–16 hours a day during the pubertal growth spurt for treating open bite cases associated with skeletal class II patterns (Mitchell, 2001). Before the growth peak begins and in the presence of a narrow maxilla, a combination of a bonded rapid maxillary expander and fixed partial appliances can effectively treat this type of malocclusion. It is essential to treat the malocclusion at an early stage and during the mixed dentition phase, to reduce the severity or eliminate the problem before the establishment of the permanent dentition.

### Permanent Dentition

Cases of mild posterior open bite in the absence of skeletal discrepancies can be treated with fixed appliances and box elastics (see Chapter 4 for elastic wear). Treatment of open bite is difficult, particularly if it has been caused by unfavourable growth leading to skeletal abnormalities. In such cases, a combination of fixed orthodontic therapy and orthognathic surgery is indicated.

### Case Study

An example of treatment of an anterior open bite in mixed dentition is shown in Figures 6.12, 6.13 and 6.14. The patient presented with the following:

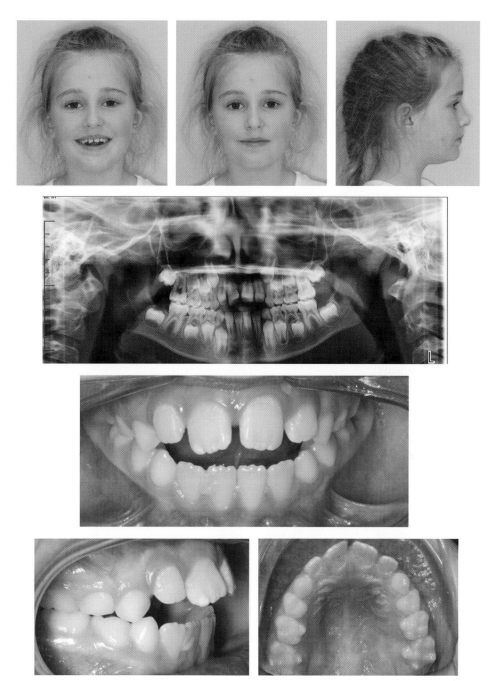

Figure 6.12  Anterior open bite in mixed dentition; initial records (courtesy of Dr Shimanto K. Purkayastha).

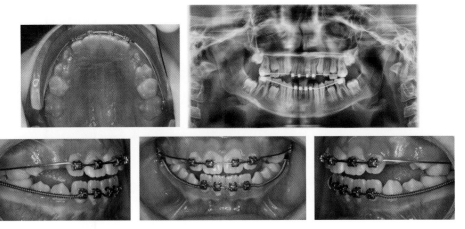

Figure 6.13 Partial braces.

- straight profile
- mesofacial
- facial symmetry
- competent lips
- anterior open bite
- class I molar relationship
- mesial step
- narrow upper arch form
- tongue-thrust swallowing pattern.

The treatment objectives were to:

- correct the open bite
- develop the upper arch form
- align and level the dental arches
- coordinate the dental arch forms
- reduce or eliminate any psychosocial issues regarding teeth and smile
- allow normal eruption of permanent teeth
- reduce the need or severity of phase II orthodontic treatment
- produce stable treatment results.

The orthodontist treated this case with the use of a non-extraction, interceptive orthopaedic development and alignment. The patient was fitted with a bonded maxillary rapid expander that was activated for a duration of about one month and left in place passively for six months as a retention. This developed the upper arch, created space for the alignment of the permanent teeth and removed unsightly buccal corridors to improve the smile aesthetics. The upper anterior segment and the lower arch were fitted with partial braces after one month of expander activation.

Upon removal of the palatal expander, the posterior teeth were bonded and the occlusion was aligned and levelled over several months with fixed appliances. After completion of the treatment, the patient was fitted with upper and lower fixed lingual retainers

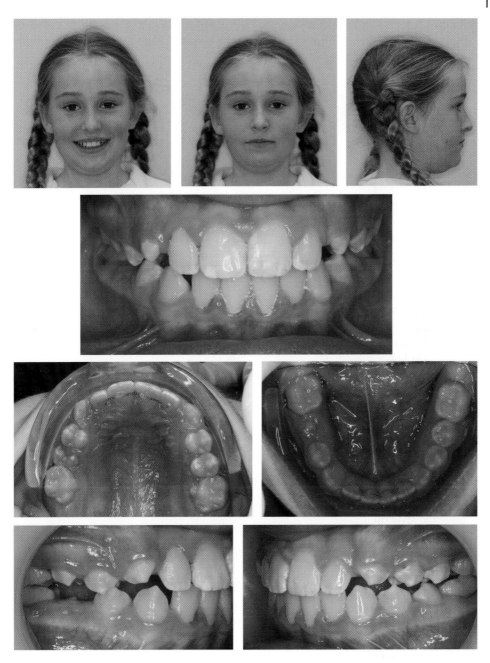

Figure 6.14 Anterior open bite in mixed dentition; final records (courtesy of Dr Shimanto K. Purkayastha).

and an upper Hawley removable retainer for nightly wear for extra retention. Recall visits were indicated to monitor tongue-thrust swallowing patterns and the eruption of the permanent dentition.

## Reference

Mitchell, L. *An Introduction to Orthodontics*. 3rd ed. Oxford: Oxford University Press; 2007.

## Further Reading

Bishara, S. E. *Textbook of Orthodontics*. Philadelphia, PA: W.B. Saunders; 2001.
Foster, T. D. *A Textbook of Orthodontics*. 3rd ed. Oxford: Blackwell Scientific; 1990.
McDonald, F., Ireland, A. J. *Diagnosis of the Orthodontic Patient*. Oxford: Oxford University Press; 1998.
Ngan, P., Fields, H. W. Open bite: a review of etiology and management. *Pediatr Dent*, 1997; 19(2): 91–98.
Ooë, T. Human Tooth and Dental Arch Development. Tokyo: Ishiyaku Publishers; 1981.

## Self-Evaluation

1 What is the term given to a tooth that cannot follow its natural eruption pattern due to a blockage of the path of eruption?
   A Dilaceration.
   B Impacted tooth.
   C Ectopic tooth.
   D Cross bite.

2 What are some of the common causes of excessive spacing?
   A Microdontia.
   B Premature tooth loss.
   C Congenitally missing teeth.
   D All of the above (a–c).

3 What appliance is commonly used as a space maintainer?
   A Transpalatal arch.
   B Twin block.
   C Bite plane.
   D Expander.

4 What is a 2 × 4 fixed appliance therapy?
   A Type of fixed appliance therapy in the permanent dentition.
   B Bonding the permanent molars and the permanent incisors.
   C Bonding the permanent molars and the permanent canines.
   D Partial fixed appliance therapy in the primary dentition.

5  What is the aim of early intervention?
   **A**  Reduce the severity of the malocclusion.
   **B**  Enhance the psychosocial wellbeing of the patient.
   **C**  Prevent complex treatments in the permanent dentition.
   **D**  All of the above.

6  Lack of spaces in the primary dentition can lead to which of the following?
   **A**  Increased overjet in the permanent dentition.
   **B**  Crowding in the permanent dentition.
   **C**  Ectopic eruptions.
   **D**  Impacted teeth.

7  Why is it critical to palpate for the permanent canines in the labial sulcus by 9–10 years of age?
   **A**  Ensure the permanent canine is present.
   **B**  Ensure it is not impacted.
   **C**  If not palpable in the sulcus, a radiographic assessment is needed.
   **D**  All of the above (a–c).

8  Which of the following appliances may be most effective for treating a child presenting with an anterior open bite and a narrow maxilla?
   **A**  Bonded rapid maxillary expander.
   **B**  Banded rapid maxillary expander.
   **C**  Bite plane.
   **D**  Face mask.

9  A posterior cross bite is mainly due to which of the following?
   **A**  Thumb sucking.
   **B**  Trauma.
   **C**  Transverse skeletal discrepancy.
   **D**  Supernumeraries.

10  Why are rapid maxillary expanders not used in very young children?
   **A**  High risk of relapse.
   **B**  Distortion to the nose.
   **C**  Expanders are contraindicated in the primary dentition.
   **D**  Due to patient discomfort.

# 7

## Treatment for Class II Malocclusion

Class II malocclusion can be corrected with a variety of treatment options, depending on how patient presents clinically and radiographically. The age and growth of the patient greatly contributes to the choice of appliance and treatment. This section briefly covers some common treatments used for class II correction and the influencing factors that can compromise a treatment. Several factors affect the specialist's choice of treatment, such as social environment, compliance, growth and facial profile; these are the determining elements in planning for the most effective treatment outcome.

## Principles of Treatment for Class II Malocclusion

Patients can present with a skeletal class II due to a maxillary excess, a mandibular deficiency, or both. If the skeletal class II is caused by maxillary excess, patients present with a backward mandibular growth rotation. This results in an increased anterior facial height. Patients with a deficient mandible typically present with a normal nasolabial angle, a smaller chin owing to a retrusive mandible, protrusion of the maxillary teeth and everted lips. The retruded position of the mandible in relation to the maxilla causes incompetent lips. In severe cases, the lower lip rests palatally to the upper incisors, resulting in minimal lip support.

   Some patients may present with a class II malocclusion and a convex profile that is caused by a dentoalveolar anomaly in the absence of an underlying skeletal discrepancy. The clinical and radiographical analysis are the key factors in differentiating the underlying problems. Generally, skeletal class II can be treated by growth modification with orthopaedic appliances in growing patients, and fixed appliance therapy with intermaxillary elastics and camouflage (extraction) treatment or orthognathic surgery in severe cases.

## Functional Appliances and Headgear

If the diagnosis is skeletal class II from a retrognathic mandible, a combination of fixed appliances and orthopaedic devices, such as a twin block, can be used in children during active growth to posture the mandible forward. Depending on the patient, the functional

*Orthodontics for Dental Hygienists and Dental Therapists*, First Edition. Tina Raked.
© 2018 John Wiley & Sons Ltd. Published 2018 by John Wiley & Sons Ltd.
Companion website: www.wiley.com/go/raked/orthodontics_dental_hygienists

appliance can be incorporated as part of phase I or phase II treatment for correction of the anteroposterior discrepancies in the jaws, while fixed appliances correct poor alignment of the teeth. The functional appliances can be used before, after or simultaneously with fixed appliances. Orthopaedic devices that are activated with facial musculature activity are called myofunctional appliances. These appliances can be fabricated in several designs to posture the mandible forward and mitigate the skeletal class II effect during an active growth phase.

Patient compliance and motivation are critically important for optimal results, particularly for removable appliances. The most suitable candidates for a functional appliance are growing patients, particularly undergoing rapid growth. The temporomandibular joint allows displacement of the condyles from the glenoid fossae. The primary goal of functional appliances is positioning the mandible downwards and forwards by increasing the endochondral growth. This is achieved via distraction to the condyles as its postured out of the glenoid fossae. Full-time or part-time (a minimum of 14–16 hours) wear of the removable appliances is highly recommended, for a duration of at least 12 months. Initially, the appliance can be uncomfortable for the patient but it is critical for practitioners to stress the importance of wearing the appliance at every review appointment, usually every six to eight weeks. Since the appliance is fitted during mixed dentition, regular adjustments may be indicated to prevent obstruction to the eruption of permanent dentition. Nightly wear of the appliance must be stressed since most growth takes place at night. Overcorrection is preferably made by orthodontists to minimise the risk of relapse. Once an active phase of treatment is completed, nightly wear of the appliance will provide adequate retention for a few months.

Functional appliances can be fixed or removable. Some can be designed with anterior capping to open the bite in cases of deep bite. Conversely, some can be fabricated with posterior capping to prevent open bites in cases with increased overjet. To fabricate these appliances, laboratory technicians require immaculate impressions with an edge-to-edge wax bite registration or digital scans of the teeth to ensure that the correct bite is captured. The bite registrations are used during fabrication to design the appliance in a manner that postures the mandible forward. Any distortions in the impressions will directly impact the fit of the appliance and this is eliminated with the use of digital scanners.

The bite registration for functional appliances differs from the bite registration taken as a record. As shown in Figure 7.1, small pieces of wax are softened in warm water and wrapped around the bite stick for the patient to bite on. The patient must bite into the

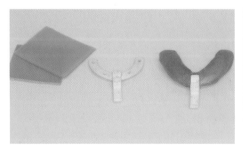 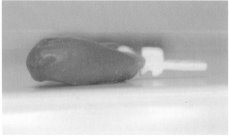

Figure 7.1 A wax bite for functional appliances.

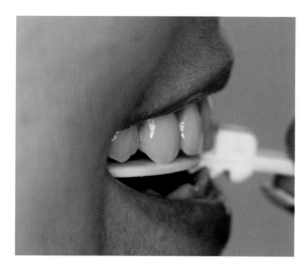

Figure 7.2  Biting edge to edge.

indentations with the upper and lower incisors biting edge to edge (Figure 7.2). Care must be taken that the patient does not posture the mandible too far forward. Every specialist would have their own unique design to the chosen functional appliance. There is a variety of appliances, some of which are described below.

### Twin Block

The twin block was introduced by William Clark in 1977. This appliance is commonly removable, although a modified fixed design is also available. It has two components: an upper and a lower block (Figure 7.3). The interlocking of the blocks in the mouth allows the forward posturing of the mandible. Full-time wear of this appliance provides a rapid optimal outcome if the patient is compliant and motivated. Twin blocks can also be designed to be worn with a headgear. Expansion of the upper arch may be needed if the patient presents with a narrow upper arch, so the upper block may be fabricated with an expansion screw in the middle to expand the upper arch and separate the palatine suture as instructed by the orthodontist.

### The Bionator

The bionator was introduced by Wilhelm Balters in 1950s. This removable orthopaedic appliance contains a single acrylic element that postures the lower incisors edge-to-edge with the upper incisors. A heavy wire loop is incorporated across the upper anterior segment. This functional appliance is designed to keep the cheeks away from the posterior teeth to allow expansion to a degree and restrict soft tissue pressure on the buccal segment. The bionator can be designed to be worn with a headgear by incorporating a face bow into the appliance (Figure 7.4).

The headgear inhibits maxillary growth as the mandible grows. This type of treatment is most effective if the patient presents with an anteroposterior maxillary excess. The headgear not only restrains the maxillary dentoalveolar structures but also acts as a great source of anchorage to prevent unwanted movement of anchor teeth (Figure 7.5).

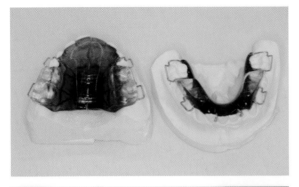

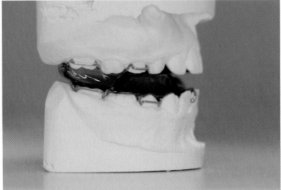

Figure 7.3 A twin block.

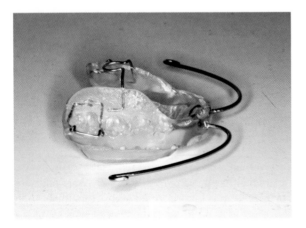

Figure 7.4 A bionator with a face bow.

If the headgear is designed as a source of anchorage it is termed extraoral anchorage. If the headgear distalises the upper permanent molars, it is termed extraoral traction. The factors that differentiates the two is the duration of wear and the force applied to either maintain the dentoalveolar structures or initiate movement. To achieve the most

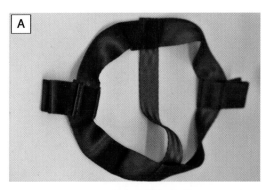

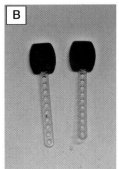
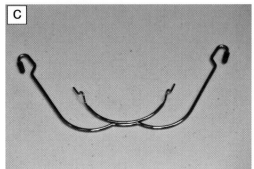

**Figure 7.5** Headgear components: A) The fabric strap that sits on the head, around the neck or a combination of the two. B) Safety strap to allow the appliance to disengage easily. C) A face bow with whisks that is usually attached to the intraoral appliance to allow attachment to the fabric and safety strap.

effective treatment outcomes with the headgear, the direction of the force may require modification throughout the treatment.

The headgear can function in three force systems, as it affects the centre of resistance of the maxillary molar in various ways (Figure 7.6):

- Cervical: a low pull as the strap rests on the neck and attaches to the bow. The force is generated below the centre of resistance of upper molars and the force created is down and back. This results in distalisation and extrusion of the upper posterior segment, allowing the mandible to rotate posteriorly backwards and downwards to open the bite. This is effective in treating class II division 2, as the molars are extruded to open the deep bite.
- Occipital: a high pull allowing the force vector to pass through or close to the centre of resistance of the upper molars. The extrusion of the molars is eliminated or minimised. This is useful in treating class II division 1, as the molars are distalised and intruded.
- A combination of cervical and occipital: a straight pull; as the vector force also passes through or close to the centre of resistance of the upper molars, it reduces or prevents extrusive forces. It applies intrusive forces to the molars.

The selection of the magnitude, direction, duration and timing of extraoral forces is determined by the specialist.

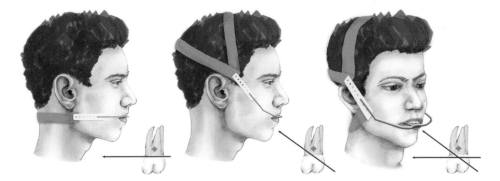

Figure 7.6 Vector and direction of force. Cervical (left): a low pull, as the strap rests on the neck and attaches to the bow; the force is generated below the centre of resistance of the upper molars. Occipital (centre): a high pull, allowing the force vector to pass through or close to the centre of resistance of the upper molars. A combination of cervical and occipital (right): a straight pull, as the vector force also passes through or close to the centre of resistance of the upper molars.

## Case Study

The patient in Figure 7.7 presented with an Angle class II division 1 malocclusion characterised by proclined maxillary incisor teeth and a retrusive mandible on a brachyfacial skeletal base. The treatment objective was an interceptive orthopaedic development. A removable functional appliance (twin block) was worn full time to address the skeletal nature of the malocclusion. The maxillary component of the appliance had a labial bow incorporated into the design to retrocline the upper incisors by wearing a headgear. Upon completion of treatment, a removable orthopaedic night-time retainer was issued for retention (Figure 7.8). The patient was kept on a recall until the permanent dentition was established to commence phase II.

### The Herbst Appliance

The Herbst appliance was introduced by Emil Herbst in 1905. It is a fixed functional appliance designed to expand the upper arch and posture the mandible forwards (Figure 7.9). The upper molars and premolars, together with the lower molars, are cemented with bands as the upper and lower jaws are connected with Herbst arms (rods). The rods may require extra activation in subsequent appointments. This is achieved by adding crimpable shims on the rods. There are also variations on how this appliance can be designed.

### The Forsus™ Appliance

The Forsus appliance is a fixed functional appliance used simultaneously with fixed appliances for treating a retrusive mandible in mild to moderate cases (Figure 7.10). Another example of a fixed class II corrector used simultaneously with fixed appliances is the powerScope. These appliances do not require laboratory set-up and are easy to install and adjust in the chair.

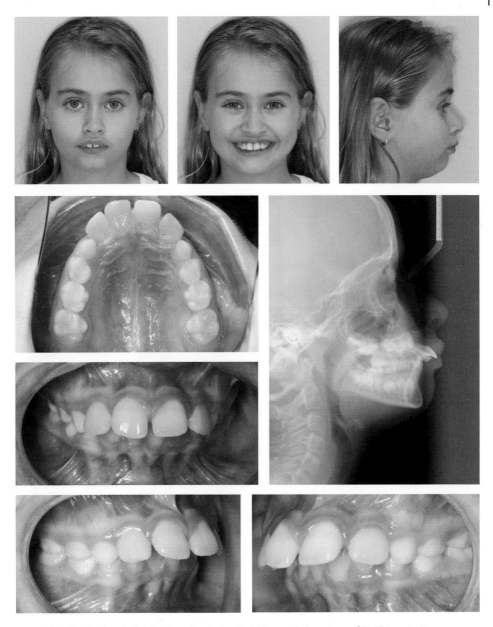

**Figure 7.7** Angle class II division 1 malocclusion; initial records (courtesy of Dr Shimanto K. Purkayastha).

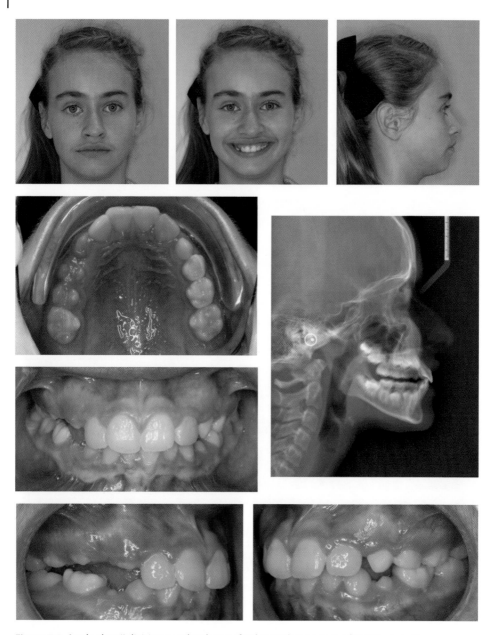

**Figure 7.8** Angle class II division 1 malocclusion; final records (courtesy of Dr Shimanto K. Purkayastha).

### Frankel Appliance

The Frankel appliance was introduced by Rolf Frankel. This appliance is also called the function regulator. Anteroposterior discrepancies of the dental arches in class II and class III can be corrected with this appliance. An acrylic lower-lip pad in the labial sulcus aids in treatment of class II division 1. Keeping the lips and cheeks away

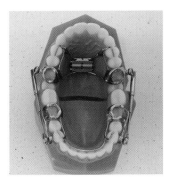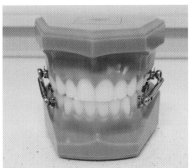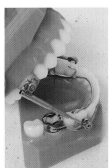

Figure 7.9  A Herbst appliance.

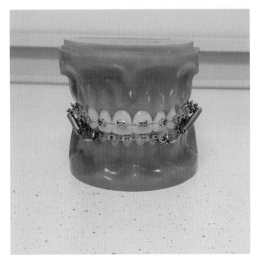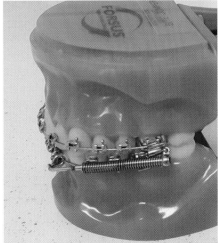

Figure 7.10  A Forsus appliance.

from the lower anterior segments allows further development of the lower labial alveolar process.

Treatment of class II division 2 is achieved with an acrylic shield in the sulcus, with an additional palatal wire to protrude the upper incisors and open the bite.

The Frankel appliance can be adapted for the treatment of class III by incorporating a labial bow to the lower incisors for retrusion. The labial acrylic shield allows some expansion by keeping the cheeks away from the buccal segments with a palatal arch incorporated in the design to protrude the upper incisors. This is type of appliance is no longer popular and is rarely used by practitioners.

## Care Instructions for Functional Appliances

The patient must be advised about how to wear the appliance (if it is removable) and it is an essential part of patient management to provide the patient with some extra time to practise wearing the appliance and ask questions as they familiarise themselves with their new appliance. Playing contact sport with removable appliances in the mouth is contraindicated. The appliance must be replaced with a mouth guard during sports and physical activity. This reduces the risk of trauma and damage. It is vital to keep the appliance clean with cold water and a toothbrush. The plate must be kept in a hard case for safe keeping. The patient must be warned that speech will be affected for a few days, although with appropriate wear of the appliance this will pass. To achieve optimum results it is essential to stress the importance of full-time wearing of the appliance to the patient and their families.

## Class II Division 1

Patients with a class II division 1 malocclusion present with increased overjet and proclined upper central incisors. Treatment of class II division 1 is crucial at an early stage as patients are more susceptible to trauma to the incisors, owing to the excessive protrusion of the upper anterior segment. The skeletal pattern can vary depending on the aetiology of the malocclusion. The most common skeletal pattern in class II is due to mandibular retrognathia (a recessive mandible). The soft tissue effect and habits can influence dentoalveolar relationships. A patient may have class I or class III skeletal patterns but habits such as digit sucking may cause proclination of the upper incisors, resulting in the development of an increased overjet.

Various techniques and combination of treatments may be used to achieve the same end result. The objective is to retract the upper incisors and to protrude the lower arch to mitigate the overjet. The orthodontist will decide on whether extractions are indicated for retraction of the upper segment by calculating the space needed for correction of the malocclusion and assessing the growth and facial profile. If the mandible is retrognathic, using functional appliances such as twin blocks aids in posturing the mandible forward in growing patients.

Another possibility is the use of a headgear with or without extractions in the upper arch. The purpose is to employ the growth of the mandible to change its position in relation to the maxilla during an active growth phase in mixed dentition. Growth can superimpose the effect during dentofacial changes (Tadic, 2007). Functional appliances will not be used beyond the growth spurt, as studies have shown that the mandible will not grow beyond its genetic potential and no further growth will be achieved in matured craniofacial structures. Thus, in severe skeletal class II cases, orthognatic surgery and fixed appliance therapy will be planned if growth has ceased. The treatment for class II division 1 involves dental and skeletal changes.

### Case Study

An example of treatment of class II division 1 is shown in Figures 7.11, 7.12 and 7.13. The patient presented with the following:

- convex profile
- brachyfacial
- incompetent lips (lip trap) from increased overjet
- class II skeletal base characterised by mandibular retrognathism
- Angle class II division 1
- class II molar relationship.

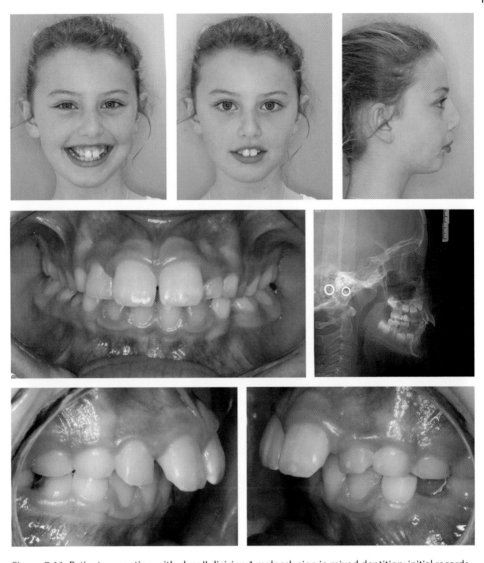

Figure 7.11 Patient presenting with class II division 1 malocclusion in mixed dentition; initial records (courtesy of Dr Shimanto K. Purkayastha).

Further findings of significance indicate a narrow maxilla and a gummy smile.

The treatment objectives for this patient were to:

- improve the facial profile
- improve the soft-tissue lip pattern
- improve the skeletal base relationship
- correct the overjet
- develop the upper arch form
- align and level the dental arches
- coordinate the dental arch forms

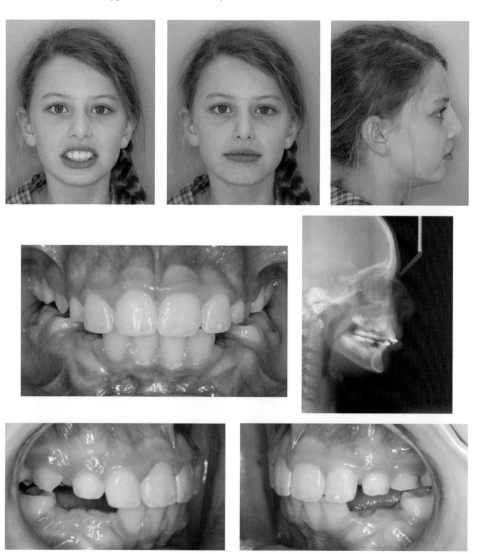

Figure 7.12 Class II division 1 malocclusion in mixed dentition; end of phase I treatment.

- establish a class I molar relationship
- establish a class I canine relationship
- reduce or eliminate any psychosocial issues regarding teeth and smile
- allow normal eruption of permanent teeth
- reduce the severity of phase II orthodontic treatment
- produce stable treatment results.

The patient was referred to the general dentist for extraction of the decayed and broken-down deciduous molar. A banded rapid maxillary expansion appliance was fitted to create sufficient space for the planned treatment and expand the maxilla. The upper and lower 2 × 4 self-ligating fixed appliances were fitted one month later, after

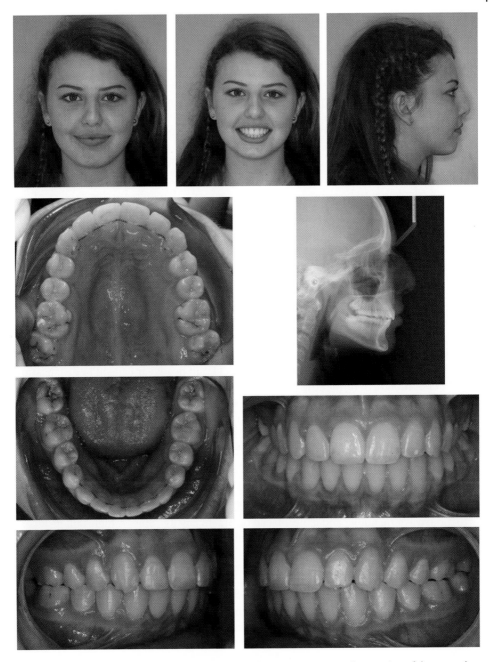

**Figure 7.13** Class II division 1 malocclusion; end of phase II treatment and correction of the premolar relationship. *Source*: Case by Dr Shimanto K Purkayastha.

sufficient expansion had been achieved. Once adequate alignment was achieved and expander removed, an orthopaedic twin block functional appliance was issued to address the skeletal nature of the malocclusion. This phase I treatment ended with a retention involving fixed lingual retainers on the upper and lower incisors, upper and lower holding arches and a night-time bionator plate. The eruption of the permanent teeth was monitored closely at recall visits.

Upon establishment of the permanent dentition, enamel wear at the premolar region was evident from an edge-to-edge bite. To correct the buccal segment, a phase II treatment of fixed appliance therapy was indicated in the upper and lower arches. The anterior fixed lingual retainers were removed to allow further correction and alignment. The duration and complexity of the treatment was dramatically reduced, as the patient had completed phase I treatment successfully and the underlying skeletal discrepancy had been corrected at an early stage. The placement of upper and lower self-ligating 0.022-inch preadjusted edgewise prescription system with selective torques provided excellent results. Delta or triangle elastic wear in the final stages of treatment allowed adequate correction to be made to the buccal segments. To increase the stability of the occlusion, the patient was fitted with upper and lower fixed lingual retainers and a nightly removable vacuum-formed retainer for retention.

## Class II Division 2

A deep overbite and brachyfacial profile are common characteristics of patients presenting with class II division 2. To correct this type of malocclusion, the deep bite must be opened up and adjusted to class II division 1 before correction. Patients with a brachyfacial profile present with a forward mandibular growth, which can be favourable once the incisal bite opening is achieved. Cervical pull headgear can aid in distalisation of the upper molars to retract the upper arch. A bite plane can also be used to allow the incisal bite opening in combination with fixed appliances.

Achieving mandibular protrusion with surgery or functional appliances causes the wider portion of the mandible to occlude on the narrow portion of the maxilla, so a maxillary expansion will accommodate this correction (Tadic, 2007).

### Mixed Dentition

In mixed dentition, a functional appliance such as a twin block is most effective in patients with a retrusive mandible and a mesofacial or brachyfacial profile. A high-pull headgear can be effective in patients with a dolichofacial profile and a retrognathic mandible.

### Permanent Dentition

A patient presenting with a mesofacial or dolichofacial profile and an excessive maxillary protrusion can be treated with fixed appliances and possibly extractions to alleviate crowding using a temporary anchorage device (see Chapter 4). Patients with a brachyfacial profile with a protrusive maxilla can be treated by distalising the upper molars with a suitable appliance using microimplants as anchorage. Mild cases can also be treated with a series of clear aligners (discussed further in Chapter 11). In severe mandibular retrognathia in mature patients whose growth has ceased, a combination of fixed orthodontic appliances and orthognathic surgery provides optimum results. Surgery may be indicated in both arches to alleviate the skeletal discrepancies.

The decision to treat a case with or without extraction requires extensive clinical investigations to determine whether the patient is a suitable case for extraction. If a case is treated with extraction, it is known as a camouflage class II because removal of teeth is employed to disguise the skeletal discrepancies. Anchorage is necessary if extractions are incorporated in the treatment, to enhance the stability of the dental arches.

Case study

An example of treatment of class II division 2 is shown in Figures 7.14, 7.15 and 7.16. The patient presented with the following:

- skeletal class II due to a retrusive mandible
- 100% overbite
- Angle class II division 2
- class II molar relationship.

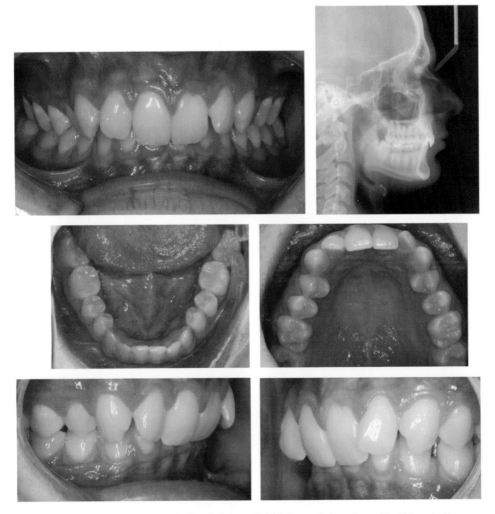

Figure 7.14 Patient presenting with class II division 2; initial records (courtesy of Dr Shimanto K. Purkayastha).

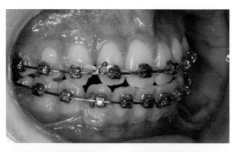

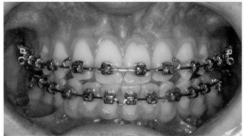 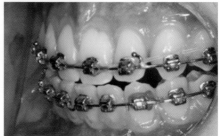

Figure 7.15 Patient presenting with class II division 2; an edge-to-edge bite is achieved using a Forsus appliance.

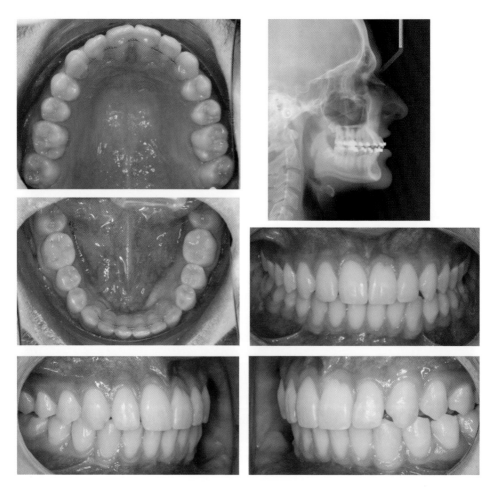

Figure 7.16 Patient presenting with class II division 2; records at the end of treatment.

The planned treatment for correction of this case was:

- placement of upper and lower fixed appliances using self-ligating 0.022-inch pread-justed edgewise prescription with selective torques to decompensate the dental arches
- use of Forsus to address the skeletal class II
- retention involving fixed lingual retainers in the upper and lower arches with a removable maxillary retainer
- monitor the development of the third molars.

The skeletal maturity of the patient, based on a radiographic hand–wrist analysis, indicated that there was some latent mandibular growth remaining, as the patient was about to enter the post-pubertal period. The patient and parent were advised that the twin block approach, given the maturing skeletal status of the patient, would not result in an anterior positioning of the mandible to the same extent as a bilateral sagittal split osteotomy (a type of orthognathic surgery described in Chapter 11).

The orthopaedic approach differs from extraction-based orthodontics by establishing an appropriate skeletal environment to accommodate all the permanent teeth. While an extraction option might result in an improvement in the appearance of the teeth, it would be to the detriment of the facial aesthetics. The facial and soft-tissue structure of some patients is such that extraction of the teeth and conventional orthodontic mechanics and space closure risks flattening the lips and accentuating the prominence of the nose and chin.

Fixed appliances allowed proclination of the upper incisors and converted the class II division 2 presentation into division 1 for the patient presented in Figure 7.14. The Forsus appliance directly addressed the structure at fault: the retrognathic mandible. The patient was fitted with fixed upper and lower lingual retainers and a removable upper vacuum-formed retainer for nightly wear for retention after treatment.

As mentioned previously, bite planes in the lower arch can aid in opening up deep bites or if an anterior cross bite of one or more teeth is present (Figure 7.17). Another method for opening deep bites is bonding bite ramps on the palatal surfaces of the

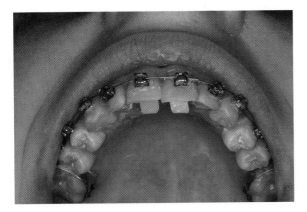

Figure 7.17  Palatal bite ramp.

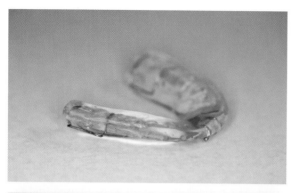

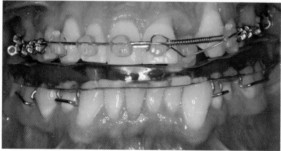

Figure 7.18 A lower bite plane used to create space between the upper and lower jaws to traction the upper left lateral incisor labially with an auxiliary wire.

upper central incisors (Figure 7.18). This is particularly helpful if the lower fixed appliances are fitted. The space that is created prevents breakage of wires or brackets from the upper teeth occluding on to the lower arch. Bite ramps can also be bonded on the occlusal surface of molars to allow slight bite opening and prevent occlusal interferences with brackets.

In summary, the objectives for treatment of class II are:

- opening up the deep bite for class II division 2
- class II correction of molars, canines and incisors
- retraction of the upper incisors or distalisation of the molars
- improving the skeletal profile by achieving a harmonious relationship between the maxilla and mandible
- freeing the lower dentoalveolus and carrying forward normal mandibular growth (orthodontic treatment can aid in reduction of the lower lip roll and retraction of the upper lip; adequate lower lip support is essential to prevent flattening of the facial profile and to preserve a satisfying lateral skeletal appearance)

If the aim of the treatment is upper retrusion, this can be achieved using:

- headgear during active growth
- insertion of microimplants for anchorage to distalise the upper arch in combination with fixed appliances
- distalising the upper arch via extractions and fixed appliance therapy.

If the aim of the treatment is lower protrusion, this can be achieved by:

• fixed functional appliances, such as Herbst, twin block, Forsus
• removable functional appliances, such a twin block in combination with a course of fixed orthodontic therapy to correct alignment and levelling of the arches
• use of class II elastics during fixed orthodontic therapy; this is a common treatment of dental class II treatment, rather than a skeletal class II.

In the case of skeletal discrepancies, a combination of therapies may be indicated. In severe cases where growth has ceased, surgery of one or both arches may be indicated with fixed orthodontic therapy.

## Reference

Tadic, N., Woods, M. Contemporary class II orthodontic and orthopaedic treatment: a review. *Aust Dent J*, 2007; 52(3): 168–174.

## Further Reading

Alexander, R. G. *The 20 Principles of the Alexander Discipline*. Hanover Park, IL: Quintessence; 2008.
Bishara, S. E. *Textbook of Orthodontics*. Philadelphia, PA: W.B. Saunders; 2001.
Foster, T. D. *A Textbook of Orthodontics*. 3rd ed. Oxford: Blackwell Scientific; 1990.
McDonald, F., Ireland, A. J. *Diagnosis of the Orthodontic Patient*. Oxford: Oxford University Press; 1998.
Mitchell, L. *An Introduction to Orthodontics*. 3rd ed. Oxford: Oxford University Press; 2007.

## Self-Evaluation

1  What is a common clinical finding of class II division 1?
   A  Increased overbite.
   B  Protrusion of the lower incisors.
   C  Deep bite.
   D  Increased overjet.

2  What is a myofunctional appliance?
   A  An appliance that postures the mandible forwards.
   B  An appliance that modifies growth before the growth spurt.
   C  Orthopaedic devices activated with facial musculature activity.
   D  All of the above (a–c).

3  Orthodontists will correct class II division 2 by first turning the occlusion into class II division 1.
   A  True.
   B  False.

4  Which of the following is NOT a functional appliance?
   **A** Frankel appliance.
   **B** Bionator.
   **C** Herbst.
   **D** Bite plane.

5  How long does the functional appliance need to be worn to achieve an effective treatment outcome?
   **A** 18 months.
   **B** 6 months.
   **C** 12 months.
   **D** 10 months.

6  Why is an expander incorporated into the upper components of some of the functional appliances?
   **A** To relieve crowding in the upper arch.
   **B** To retrude the upper incisors.
   **C** To expand the upper arch as the mandible is protruded the narrow portion of the maxilla will be contacting the wider portion of the mandible.
   **D** All of the above (a–c).

7  Which of the following is a fixed functional appliance?
   **A** Bionator.
   **B** Forsus.
   **C** Twin block.
   **D** Function regulator.

8  Why are functional appliances only used during active growth?
   **A** No further growth will be achieved in matured patients.
   **B** Functional appliances are only designed for growth modification.
   **C** After the growth spurt the mandible will not grow beyond its genetic potential.
   **D** All of the above.

9  Backward mandibular growth is unfavourable for treatment of class II division 1.
   **A** True.
   **B** False.

10  Which of the following plates is ideal for incisal bite opening in combination with fixed appliances?
   **A** Twin block.
   **B** Bite plane.
   **C** Hawley retainer.
   **D** Bionator.

# 8

# Treatment for Class III Malocclusion

Class III malocclusion is characterised by mandibular prognathism, maxillary retrognathia or both. Patients typically present with a concave profile because of a prominent mandible. Some common dental concerns associated with class III malocclusion are:

- narrow maxillary arch
- broad mandible
- crowding
- posterior and anterior cross bite.

The soft tissue has minimal aetiological effect in class III patients. The degree of anteroposterior and vertical skeletal discrepancies determines the complexity of the necessary treatment. Unfavourable growth greatly affects the treatment outcome and highly increases the risk of relapse following treatment. A better prognosis is evident in patients who are able to achieve an edge-to-edge incisor relationship, which is also known as pseudo-class III.

Treatment options for class III malocclusion vary, depending on the location of the excess or deficiency (Guyer et al., 1986). Mandibular prognathism or overgrowth with a normal maxilla is known as true mandibular prognathism. Hypoplastic maxilla results in an anterior cross bite in the absence of mandibular prognathism. A combination of maxillary retrusion and mandibular protrusion is one of the most commonly seen patterns in skeletal class III malocclusions.

## Treatment in Mixed Dentition

The use of an acrylic splint expander (a bonded rapid maxillary expander) simultaneously together with a face mask (reverse pull headgear) is an effective treatment option for skeletal class III malocclusions during an active growth phase. This type of treatment was introduced by McNamara. The expansion of the maxilla aids in correction of the narrow upper arch and eliminates any posterior cross bite. The bonded rapid maxillary expander (RME) is designed with vestibular hooks to allow the attachment of the facemask for protraction of the maxilla (Figure 8.1). The facemask must be worn for a

*Orthodontics for Dental Hygienists and Dental Therapists*, First Edition. Tina Raked.
© 2018 John Wiley & Sons Ltd. Published 2018 by John Wiley & Sons Ltd.
Companion website: www.wiley.com/go/raked/orthodontics_dental_hygienists

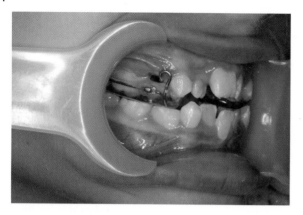

Figure 8.1 Vestibular J hook incorporated in the design of a bonded rapid maxillary expander for wearing with a face mask.

minimum of 14–16 hours for optimal results. For better patient comfort, this appliance is recommended to be worn outside of school hours. The degree of activation of the palatal expander is decided by the orthodontist. The treatment goal is to move the maxilla downwards and forwards using the face mask. Thus, when the face mask hooks are adjusted for elastic wear, it is critical to ensure that the elastics pull the maxilla downwards and forwards (Figure 8.2). This type of treatment is shown to be more effective in patients with mild to moderate skeletal class III malocclusions with a hyperdivergent growth pattern and a retrognathic maxilla.

Congenital class III malocclusions deteriorate after the growth spurt and surgery might be indicated. Thus, treatment might need to be delayed until growth has ceased to prevent relapse. Depending on the position of the maxilla in relation to the craniofacial reference points, the choice of the surgical procedure will vary (discussed further in Chapter 11).

Early intervention in some patients is advantageous for several reasons, although the timing and duration of the treatment is solely decided by the orthodontist. The objective of early treatment is:

- to reduce the severity of the problem, thus reducing the complexity of phase II treatment
- to enhance a functional occlusion
- to improve the psychosocial wellbeing of the patient
- to create favourable dentofacial development that accommodates future growth
- to reduce the need for future orthognathic surgery, although it is important to raise patient awareness that surgery may be indicated despite the success of the treatment. This possibility will depend on the type and degree of further growth.

The Frankel III regulator is not a popular appliance, although it has been used to treat some skeletal class III malocclusions. This functional appliance aids in forward

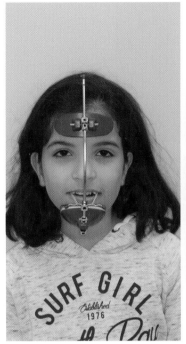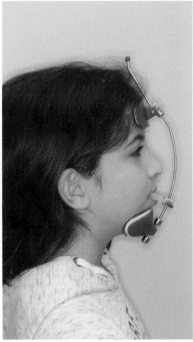

**Figure 8.2** Face mask with elastics at a downward angle to protract the maxilla downwards and forwards.

development of the maxilla by using muscle force and redirects mandibular growth posteriorly. The labial pads distance the upper lip from the maxilla and allow the force to be transferred to the mandible as the appliance closely fits in the lower arch. This appliance is only effective with good patient compliance and full-time wear of the appliance. Chin cup therapy was another effective treatment in patients with skeletal class III malocclusion who presented with a normal maxillary position. This early intervention inhibited mandibular growth in mild to moderate cases. This type of treatment is also no longer popular, particularly with the increased availability of treatments involving temporary anchorage devices and skeletal plates. Incorporation of temporary anchorage devices in skeletal class III treatment can be achieved in many ways and these devices have proven to be one of the most effective treatment options for class III malocclusions; for example, using lower skeletal plates in combination with an RME supported by a temporary anchorage device.

## Case Studies

An example of treating a class III malocclusion using skeletal plates and an RME supported by a temporary anchorage device is seen in Figures 8.3–8.6.

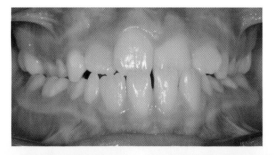

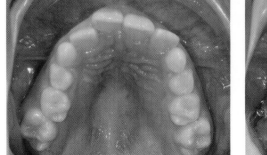
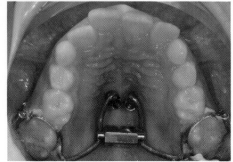

Figure 8.3 Insertion of a rapid maxillary anchorage device with a super screw supported by a temporary anchorage device for treatment of class III with an ovoid upper arch. *Source*: Case by Dr Nour Eldin Tarraf.

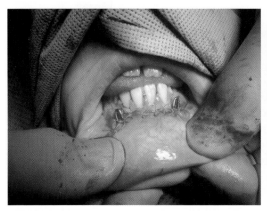
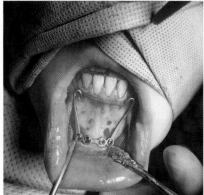

Figure 8.4 Surgical insertion of skeletal plates. *Source*: Case by Dr Adit Bahl.

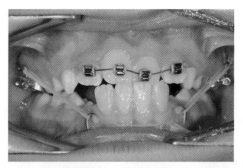

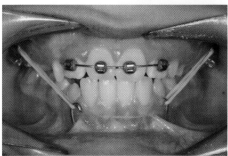
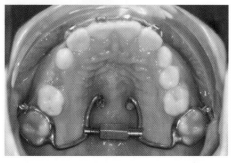

**Figure 8.5** Correction of anterior cross bite with elastic wear from the skeletal plate to the rapid maxillary expander. Active self-ligating brackets are used on the upper incisors to correct crowding.

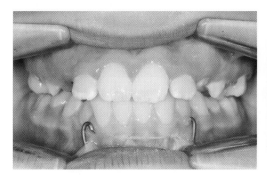
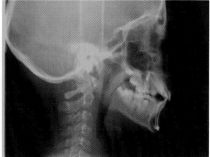

**Figure 8.6** Correction of a class III malocclusion.

Another example of treating class III in mixed dentition is seen in Figures 8.7 and 8.8. The patient presented with the following:

- brachyfacial
- concave profile
- competent lips
- symmetrical face
- class III incisor relationship with retroclined upper incisors
- molar relationships: right side, class III; left side, class II
- narrow upper arch
- bilateral cross bite.

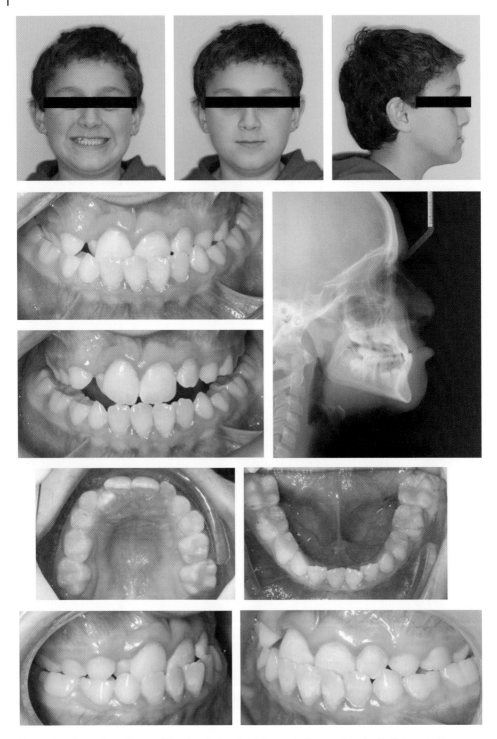

**Figure 8.7** Correction of a class III malocclusion; initial records. *Source*: Case by Dr Shimanto K. Purkayastha.

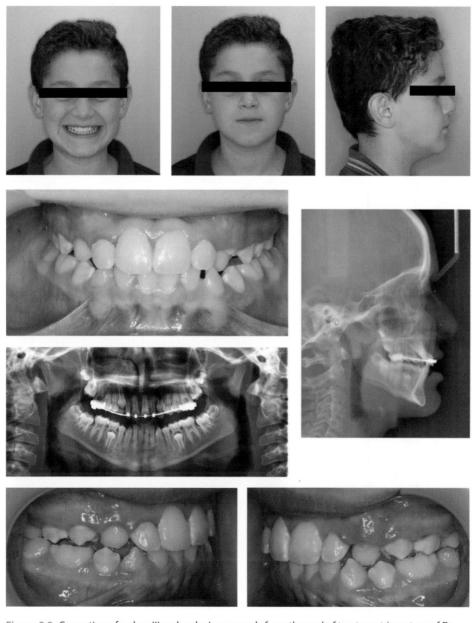

Figure 8.8 Correction of a class III malocclusion; records from the end of treatment (courtesy of Dr Shimanto K. Purkayastha).

The orthodontic diagnosis revealed an Angle class III malocclusion which displays a centric relation and centric occlusion discrepancy with an anterior functional shift of the mandible with bilateral posterior palatal cross bite. The chosen treatment plan was an interceptive orthopaedic development of the maxilla:

- Using a rapid maxillary expansion with vestibular hooks for attachment of the face mask, to:
  ○ develop the upper arch

- ○ correct posterior cross bite
- ○ create space for the alignment of the permanent teeth
- ○ remove unsightly buccal corridors to improve smile aesthetics.
- Placement of upper 2 × 4 fixed self-ligating appliances with 0.022-inch pre-adjusted edgewise prescription with selective torques.
- Retention involving maxillary fixed lingual retainers for the upper incisors and a maxillary removable retainer.
- Review the eruption of the permanent dentition.
- Review mandibular growth.

This orthopaedic approach differs from extraction-based orthodontics by establishing an appropriate skeletal environment to accommodate all the permanent teeth. Instead of extracting teeth to create space in a deficient jaw, dentofacial orthopaedics alters the bony housing to accommodate all the permanent teeth. While an extraction option may result in an improvement in the appearance of the teeth, it would not be beneficial to the aesthetics of the facial profile. Extraction of the teeth in this case runs the risk of flattening the lips, accentuating the nose and chin prominence – characteristics associated with increased age.

The patient was compliant with the face mask and it functioned well by directing an anterior and inferior force on the sutures of the retrognathic maxilla, thereby stimulated its growth and addressing the skeletal component of the malocclusion. Anchorage for the face mask was provided by a bonded RME appliance. This latter appliance disrupted the maxillary sutural system once it was activated so the effectiveness of the face mask (in terms of skeletal movement) was enhanced.

For it to be effective, the ideal time for facemask treatment is before 10–11 years of age. Beyond this age, increased interdigitation of the circumaxillary sutures makes skeletal movement harder to achieve.

Once sufficient space was gained, the upper incisors were bonded with passive self-ligating brackets and the face mask was reduced to nightly wear after six months of part-time wear. Once the bonded RME was removed, the face mask was no longer worn and the posterior teeth were bonded with self-ligating brackets. This bracket system is the combination of passive self-ligating brackets, high-technology arch wires and simplified treatment protocols that work together in a low-friction and low-force system that is clinically proven to provide remarkable outcomes.

Once the appropriate alignment was achieved by the orthodontist, fixed lingual retainers were fitted in the upper arch and the patient was given a Hawley retainer for nightly wear. The eruption of the permanent dentition was monitored closely in regular reviews. Patient and parent are warned that subsequent adverse growth may lead to the redevelopment of a class III malocclusion, for which an orthognathic solution at the end of growth would be considered.

## Treatment in Permanent Dentition

If the patient presents with a class III molar relationship with mild skeletal discrepancies, the treatment objective is correction of the anterior and posterior occlusal relationships. These cases can be treated with a combination of fixed orthodontic therapy and intermaxillary class III elastics. Depending on where the deficiency or excess exists and the degree of discrepancy, orthodontists can decide on a camouflage treatment or a combination of orthodontics and surgical correction. Camouflage is an extraction-based treatment plan using dentoalveolar compensatory mechanisms to correct the malocclusion.

An example of a class III correction in an adult patient whose growth had ceased, using a combination of orthodontics and orthognathic surgery, is seen in Figures 8.9 and 8.10. The patient presented with the following:

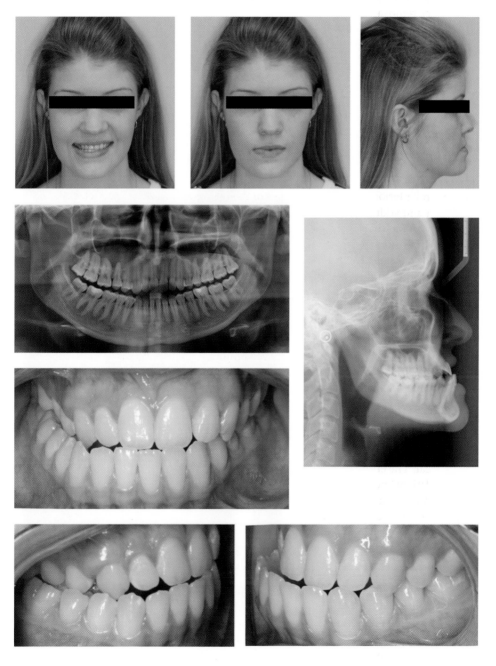

**Figure 8.9** Correction of a class III malocclusion in an adult; initial records. *Source*: Case by Dr Shimanto K. Purkayastha.

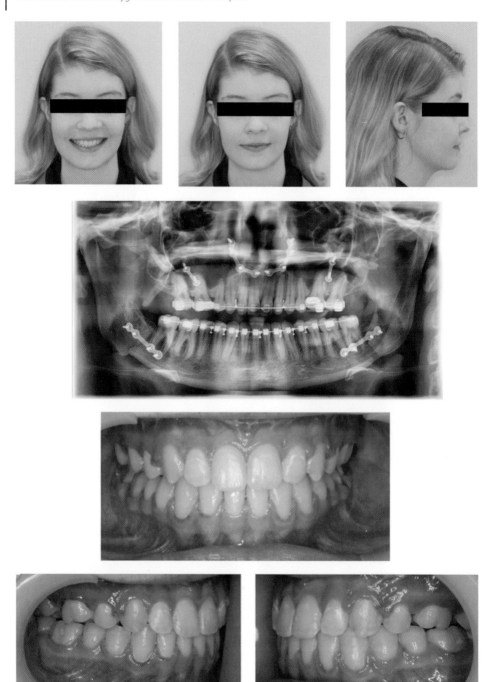

Figure 8.10 Correction of a class III malocclusion in an adult; final records (courtesy of Dr Shimanto K. Purkayastha).

- concave profile with a maxillary deficiency
- facial asymmetry
- mandibular deviation to the right
- class III incisor and molar relationships
- bilateral posterior palatal cross bite.

The Angle class III malocclusion was bimaxillary in nature (maxillary deficiency and a mandibular excess) with a component of mandibular asymmetry. The severity of the malocclusion meant that the patient became a suitable candidate for a combined orthodontic orthognathic surgical approach.

The presurgical objective was placement of the maxillary and mandibular fixed appliances to decompensate the dental arches. The cephalometric analysis indicated a considerable protraction of the maxillary anterior teeth. The upper first premolars were extracted to remove this dentoalveolar compensation and to retract the maxillary anterior segment, thereby worsening the class III malocclusion to allow sufficient underbite to correct the skeletal imbalance. A bimaxillary surgery of Le Fort I advancement of the maxilla (see Chapter 11) and an asymmetric setback of the mandible was chosen for the surgical correction. The extractions of the first premolars and the third molars took place after placement of a maxillary holding arch to preserve the anchorage, to allow sufficient retraction of the maxillary anterior segment. Once the dentoalveolar decompensation was achieved, the surgery took place. The treatment completed with final detailing of the arches and elastic wear to stabilise the occlusion. The upper and lower anterior teeth were bonded with fixed lingual retainers and a nightly removable vacuum formed retainer was issued for additional retention.

## Summary

In summary, the objectives of class III treatments are as follows:

- Proclination of the upper arch if the patient presents with an anterior cross bite, class I skeletal profile or a mild class III skeletal profile. In children with mixed dentition, protraction of the upper arch is achieved using a bonded RME with a face mask or incorporation of temporary anchorage device and skeletal plates as part of the treatment.
- Mild to moderate class III can be treated by reclining the lower labial segment with or without upper proclination. This can be achieved using fixed appliances and elastic wear. Space can be created with round or rectangular arch wires but if the arch is not naturally spaced, extractions may be indicated.
- For severe class III, surgery is indicated after growth has ceased and further dental corrections are made with fixed appliances.

Several factors influence the decision on the type of treatment used for correction of class III malocclusions, such as:

- the degree of reverse jet
- the position of the maxilla

- the position of the mandible
- the vertical excess
- the angulation of the incisors in both dental arches

The higher the skeletal discrepancy, the lower the chances of treating patients with orthodontics alone.

## Reference

Guyer, E. C., Ellis, E. E., McNamara, J. A., et al. Components of class III malocclusion in Juveniles and adolescents. *Angle Orthod*, 1986. 56(1): 7–30.

## Further Reading

Bishara, S. E. *Textbook of Orthodontics*. Philadelphia, PA: W.B. Saunders; 2001.

Foster, T. D. *A Textbook of Orthodontics*. 3rd ed. Oxford: Blackwell Scientific; 1990.

McDonald, F., Ireland, A. J. *Diagnosis of the Orthodontic Patient*. Oxford: Oxford University Press; 1998.

Mitchell, L. *An Introduction to Orthodontics*. 3rd ed. Oxford: Oxford University Press; 2007.

Park, J. U., Baik, S. H. Classification of angle class III malocclusion and its treatment modalities. *Int J Adult Orthod*, 2001; 16(1): 19–29.

## Self-Evaluation

1 Which of the following is considered to be one of the best treatment options for correction of a moderate skeletal class III due to a retrognathic maxilla and a hyperdivergent growth pattern in mixed dentition?
   A Fixed appliances.
   B Bonded rapid maxillary expander and face mask.
   C Head gear.
   D Extractions and fixed appliances.

2 What is a pseudo-class III?
   A A class III patient who can posture the mandible posteriorly to achieve an edge-to-edge bite.
   B Protruded lower incisors and retruded upper incisors.
   C An edge-to-edge bite that slides into a class III malocclusion.
   D Protrusive mandible.

3 How can a skeletal class III patient present?
   A mandibular prognathism or overgrowth with a normal maxilla.
   B retrusive maxilla and a protruded mandible.
   C Hypoplastic maxilla resulting in an anterior cross bite.
   D All of the above (a–c).

4 Which plate is most effective in correction of the anterior cross bite in combination with fixed appliances with minimal skeletal discrepancy?
   A  Bite plane.
   B  Frankel appliance.
   C  Herbst appliance.
   D  Bionator.

5 What are some of the advantages of early treatment of class III malocclusion?
   A  Improve the patient's psychosocial wellbeing.
   B  Achieve an aesthetic and functional occlusion.
   C  Reduce the complexity of the orthodontic problem.
   D  All of the above (a–c).

6 The type of surgery for class III treatment is dependent upon which of the following?
   A  The patient's age.
   B  The patient's compliance.
   C  The position of the maxilla and mandible in relation to the craniofacial reference points.
   D  a and c.

7 What are the minimum hours necessary for face mask wear to achieve optimum results?
   A  2–3 hours a day.
   B  4–6 hours a day.
   C  10 hours a day.
   D  14–16 hours a day.

8 A better prognosis is evident in patients who are able to achieve an edge-to-edge incisor relationship.
   A  True.
   B  False.

9 Which factor most determines the complexity of class III treatment?
   A  The degree of anteroposterior malrelation.
   B  Vertical skeletal discrepancy.
   C  The degree of crowding.
   D  Where the deficiency or excess exists.

10 What is the most common facial profile seen in skeletal class III patients?
   A  Convex.
   B  Concave.
   C  Bimaxillary.
   D  Straight.

9

# Treatment for Cleft Palate

This chapter provides a brief summary of the palate development and the craniofacial anomaly associated with the lip and palate. The depth of cleft palate and cleft treatment is beyond the scope of this textbook. However, a brief summary will aid in creating a better understanding of this aspect of orthodontics.

## Palate Formation

The completion of the palate takes up to 12 weeks in utero and initiated by the sixth week of pregnancy. Two events occur for the maxilla to be structured:

1) Development of the maxillary alveolar process and the primary palate formation. The primary palate (also known as the premaxilla) is located anterior to the incisive foramen. These structures form the body of the maxilla. The medial and lateral nasal processes fuse with the maxillary processes.
2) Formation of the secondary palate as the lateral palatine shelves elevate and fuse (Figure 9.1). The secondary palate is located posterior to the incisive foramen and gives rise to the soft and hard palates. Any disturbances at this stage may cause a defect in the fusion of the plates and may result in a cleft palate.

Cleft lip and cleft palate are two distinct defects that commonly occur concomitantly (Figure 9.2). These defects occur when the merging between mesenchymal connective tissues during the embryonic development miscarries, resulting in malformation of the lip and/or the palate. If the medial nasal process fails to fuse with the maxillary process, a cleft in the lip develops which may be unilateral or bilateral (Figure 9.3). If the lip is only affected by this deformity, generally there are minimal dental concerns, although it may involve the alveolar process. A cleft in the palate can affect the alveolus, leading to other dental defects. Examples of the dental anomalies associated with cleft palate include hypodontia, hyperdontia, delayed eruption and enamel defects such as enamel hypoplasia. The shape of the cleft also affects the eruption pattern and alignment of the teeth.

*Orthodontics for Dental Hygienists and Dental Therapists*, First Edition. Tina Raked.
© 2018 John Wiley & Sons Ltd. Published 2018 by John Wiley & Sons Ltd.
Companion website: www.wiley.com/go/raked/orthodontics_dental_hygienists

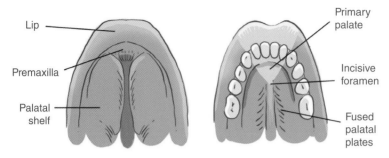

Figure 9.1 Formation of the palate.

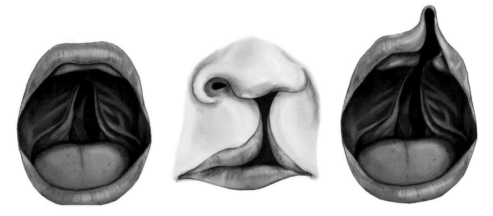

Figure 9.2 Cleft palate (left); cleft lip (centre); cleft palate and lip (right).

## Treatment of Cleft Palate

Treatment of cleft palate involves a team of healthcare professionals working together, such as plastic surgeons, paediatrician, ear, nose and throat specialists, oral maxillofacial surgeons, orthodontists, nutritionists and speech pathologists. The complexity of the treatment depends on the severity of the malformation. Cleft palate is associated with airway obstruction, feeding disorders and otitis media (middle ear infection; Wiet and Biavati, 2015). It is therefore essential that all affected systems are treated. Treatment may be necessary at various stages throughout the patient's life, depending on the severity and complexity of the craniofacial deformity.

Nutritionists provide dietary guidance to families to ensure newborns with a cleft palate receive sufficient nutrition. Speech pathologists carry out special feeding training for children who have difficulty feeding because of a complete cleft of the lip and palate or a very extensive cleft palate. Since there is a lack of a distinct barrier between the nasal floor and the oral environment, feeding is difficult for these patients, which results in distress for their families as well as for the patients. This is particularly difficult in neonates, as the milk travels through the nasal cavity. Prosthodontists or orthodontists

A B

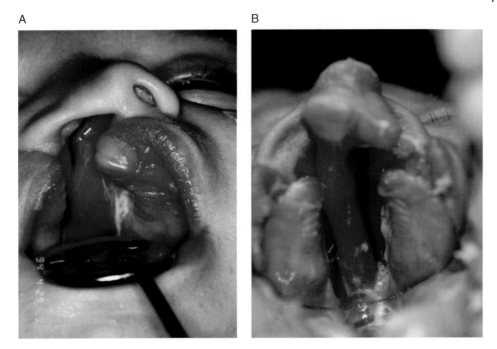

Figure 9.3 A cleft lip may be unilateral A) or bilateral B).

will provide feeding plates that can alleviate the problem. To improve the eruption of the teeth in the early stages and prior to orthodontic alignment, bone grafting of the alveolar defect may be indicated.

## Case Study

The patient in Figure 9.4 was born with a narrow premaxilla and a complete cleft lip and palate on the left side. The eruption of the dentition was monitored closely and treatment commenced in the early mixed dentition. The orthodontic diagnosis was a class III malocclusion with a missing permanent upper left lateral incisor. The maxillary expansion was carried out to address the narrow maxilla and alveolar bone was grafted in the left alveolar cleft region to allow the eruption of the permanent upper left canine. The canine was surgically exposed and bonded with a chain to traction it labially. Owing to its palatal position, this was not possible, which lead to surgical extraction of the tooth. The upper right first premolar, lower right second premolar and the lower left first premolar were extracted for orthodontic correction and alignment, as the option of orthognathic surgery was declined by the patient. The upper left first premolar was mesialised into the canine space and an implant was placed for the congenitally missing upper left lateral incisor upon completion of the orthodontic treatment.

The treatment of cleft cases is complicated and lengthy, and thus requires the attention and cooperation of many specialists.

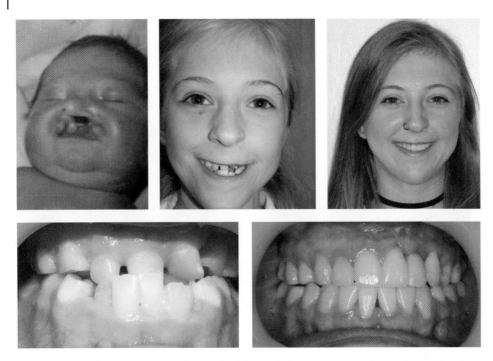

Figure 9.4 Complete cleft lip and palate on the left side: before and after treatment. *Source*: Case by by Dr Kit Chan.

## Reference

Wiet, G. J. Biavati, M. J., Rocha-Worley, G. Reconstructive surgery for cleft palate treatment and management. Medscape, 17 August 2015. Available at http://emedicine. medscape.com/article/878062-treatment (accessed 7 April 2017).

## Further Reading

Bishara, S. E. *Textbook of Orthodontics*. Philadelphia, PA: W.B. Saunders; 2001.

Brand, R. W., Isselhard, D. E. *Anatomy of Orofacial Structures: A comprehensive approach*. 7th ed. St Louis, MO: Elsevier Mosby.

Burstone, C. J., Marcotte, M. E. *Problem Solving in Orthodontics: Goal-Oriented Treatment Strategies*. Hanover Park, IL: Quintessence; 2000.

Chiego, D. J. *Essentials of Oral Histology and Embryology: A clinical approach*. 4th ed. St Louis, MO: Elsevier Mosby; 2014.

Foster, T. D. *A Textbook of Orthodontics*. 3rd ed. Oxford: Blackwell Scientific; 1990.

Goose, D. H., Appleton, J. *Human Dentofacial Growth*. Oxford: Pergamon Press; 1982.

McDonald, F., Ireland, A. J. *Diagnosis of the Orthodontic Patient*. Oxford: Oxford University Press; 1998.

Mitchell, L. *An Introduction to Orthodontics*. 3rd ed. Oxford: Oxford University Press; 2007.

Ooë, T. *Human Tooth and Dental Arch Development*. Tokyo: Ishiyaku Publishers; 1981.

Ranly, D. M. (ed.) *A Synopsis of Craniofacial Growth*. Norwalk, CT: Appleton and Lange; 1988.

Welbury, R. R., Duggal, M. S., Hosey, M. T. *Paediatric Dentistry*. 4th ed. Oxford: Oxford University Press; 2012.

## Self-Evaluation

1   Cleft lip and cleft palate are considered to be one anomaly.
   **A** True.
   **B** False.

2   Which practitioners need to be involved in treatment of cleft lip and palate?
   **A** Orthodontist.
   **B** Oral maxillofacial surgeon.
   **C** Speech pathologist and nutritionists.
   **D** All of the above (a–c).

3   What procedure aids in eruption of teeth?
   **A** Orthognathic surgery.
   **B** Extractions.
   **C** Bone grafting.
   **D** Orthodontic alignment.

4   Why does cleft palate result in eating disorders?
   **A** The lack of a distinct barrier between the nasal floor and the oral environment makes feeding difficult.
   **B** Lack of lip support makes eating difficult.
   **C** Position of the teeth can be affected by the cleft palate, therefore chewing can be difficult.
   **D** Because of the size of the tongue.

5   Cleft lip and cleft palate are congenital disorders occurring during the initial development stages.
   **A** True.
   **B** False.

6   What are some of the common clinical dental concerns in patients with cleft lip and palate?
   **A** Hyperdontia.
   **B** Hypodontia.
   **C** Enamel defects.
   **D** All of the above (a–c).

7 Otitis media is commonly seen in patients with cleft lip and palate.
   A True.
   B False.

8 There are minimal dental defects in patients with a cleft lip.
   A True.
   B False.

9 Cleft lip and palate can only occur bilaterally.
   A True.
   B False.

10 What are some of the common complications associated with this deformity?
   A Eating disorder.
   B Airway obstruction.
   C Otitis media.
   D All of the above (a–c).

# 10

# Retention

The completion of a course of orthodontic treatment is followed by a stabilisation phase, which is known as retention. The objective is to prevent relapse, which is loss of orthodontic correction and movement of the teeth from the ideal aesthetic and functional position. During orthodontic therapy, the periodontal ligaments stretch and reorganise to accommodate the movement of the socket and to make tooth movement possible. If the teeth are not stabilised in their socket, the fibres of the periodontal ligaments will contract and relapse will occur. Relapse is multifactorial. Some contributing factors are continuous growth and muscular imbalances after active orthodontic treatment has ceased. Failing to eliminate the aetiology of the initial malocclusion is associated with relapse as well; for example, persistent digit sucking after completion of an orthodontic treatment will result in recurrence of an open bite. Studies prove that long-term retention is beneficial for patients and reduces post-treatment relapse. Over the years, there have been several interpretations of relapse and retention. Some commonly used retentions are discussed in this chapter, although retention is customised for each individual by the orthodontist and can greatly vary.

## Importance of Retention

Retention is necessary for the following reasons:

- to allow newly formed bone (osteoid) to mature
- allow gingival fibres and periodontal ligaments to reorganise and adapt to the new arrangements
- neuromuscular adaptation
- to reduce the negative effects of continuous growth on the new occlusion to a degree
- to enhance the stability of orthodontic correction after completion of active treatment.

Orthodontists plan retention during the initial stages of treatment and discuss it with the patient before treatment starts. As with orthodontic treatment, the decision on the type and duration of retention varies among orthodontists. The type of retention planned is highly dependent upon growth, periodontal health, the initial malocclusion, the type of treatment and the condition of the soft tissues. It can take up to six months for the periodontal ligaments to reorganise and adapt to the new position and secure

*Orthodontics for Dental Hygienists and Dental Therapists*, First Edition. Tina Raked.
© 2018 John Wiley & Sons Ltd. Published 2018 by John Wiley & Sons Ltd.
Companion website: www.wiley.com/go/raked/orthodontics_dental_hygienists

the tooth in the newly positioned socket (Mitchell, 2001). It also takes up to six months for the collagenous fibres in the gingiva to reorganise. However, some gingival fibres, such as the elastic supracrestal fibres, have a prolonged reorganisation time, which can take up to 12 months after removal of appliances. Therefore, retention is indicated for at least six months or longer post treatment. Studies prove that circumferential supracrestal fiberotomy a few weeks before removal of appliances can prevent significant relapse. This is particularly effective in cases of severe rotation.

Once phase I treatment is completed during mixed dentition, retention is recommended until the permanent dentition is established. Permanent retention is critical for prevention of relapse in poor periodontal conditions, as teeth will drift. It may be difficult to guarantee the permanence of the orthodontic correction for every treatment; however, orthodontists consider several factors and carefully plan retention to achieve as much stability of the end results as possible.

## Fixed Retainers

Fixed retainers are micromechanically bonded flexible multistranded wires or rigid stainless steel wires across the palatal and lingual surfaces of the anterior teeth (Figure 10.1). In some cases, buccal fixed retainers can be used and these are more commonly used in the posterior region for better aesthetics. The rigid stainless steel is only secured at either end on the canines to ensure that it is passive. Active fixed retainers induce unwanted tooth movement. This type of retention is widely used after completion of a course of phase I and phase II fixed orthodontic therapy.

Generally, fixed retainers can be left in place permanently to avoid any post-treatment relapse. Fixed retainers cause minimal or no discomfort for the patient. Once

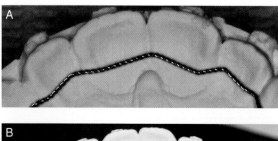

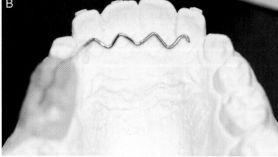

Figure 10.1  A) Flexible multistranded wires. B) V-loop to allow better access for flossing.

the orthodontist confirms the ideal root and crown position on the final radiographs, upper and lower impressions or digital scans of the teeth are required for fabrication of fixed retainers. Even if one arch requires a fixed retainer, upper and lower impressions are needed as laboratory technicians need both arches for articulation of the plaster models to make sure the fabricated fixed retainers do not cause premature contacts.

These fixed retainers can make oral hygiene and maintenance difficult and impact interproximal cleaning or flossing. Patients must be advised to use super floss to achieve adequate interproximal cleaning.

## Bonding Fixed Retainers

Steps involved in bonding fixed lingual or palatal retainers are shown in Box 10.1.

**Box 10.1  Bonding Fixed Lingual or Palatal Retainers**

Bonding Fixed Lingual or Palatal Retainers Box 10.1

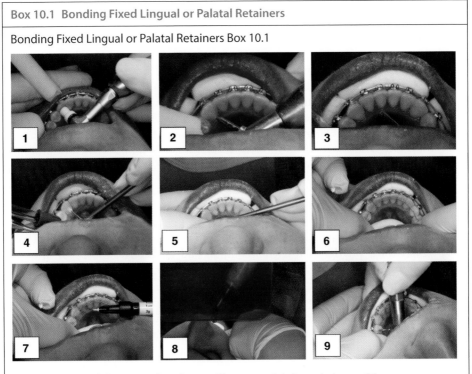

1) Prophylaxis of the enamel surfaces will remove debris and plaque (1).
2) For better retention, the enamel surfaces are mircoetched with aluminium oxide (2). The enamel surfaces must be rinsed thoroughly and dried (3).
3) Orthophosphoric acid 37% is used for at least 15 seconds (4) and washed with water thoroughly (sufficient isolation is critical to prevent saliva contamination and weak bonding, thus use of cheek and tongue retractors is essential).
4) Once a frosty etched enamel appearance is achieved upon drying, a thin layer of bond is placed over the prepared enamel surfaces and set with a curing light (5).

5) The retainers that are premade in the dental laboratory are usually fabricated with some form of an additional support to allow easy handling and better fixation of the retainer against the teeth (6). Another useful method is to use floss to secure the retainer tightly against the tooth.

6) Composite resin is used in increments over the retainers (7). Ensure that the retainer is firmly secured against the tooth before curing the composite (8). It is also critical to ensure that sufficient composite resin covers the wire and the tooth surface.

7) All rough surfaces must be removed and polished to prevent trauma to the soft tissues (9).

8) It is essential to ensure that the fixed lingual retainers do not cause premature contacts. The occlusion must be assessed using articulating paper.

## Removable Retainers

The two most commonly used removable retainers are Hawley plates and vacuum-formed thermo retainers. These retainers can be designed for upper or lower arches, or both. Full-time wear or nightly wear of the retainer, design and duration of retention are decided by the specialist. Fixed retainers can be used in combination with nightly wear of a removable retainer. Orthodontists may recommend full-time wear of a passive removable retainer for a duration of about three to six months and eventually reduce it to nightly wear with or without fixed retainers. Upon completion of a course of a functional appliance therapy, typically, nightly wear of the appliance will suffice until the rate of growth has reduced. There are several ways in which retention can be planned and the objective and goal of the orthodontist can vary, depending on their training and experience. Growth and facial changes are always considered in children and adolescents.

### Hawley Plates

There are active and passive components to Hawley retainers. The acrylic base is a cold-cured resin which provides sufficient retention and anchorage. Clasps, such as the Adams clasp or ball clasp, are incorporated into the appliance to enhance the retention and stability between the acrylic portion of the plate, teeth and soft tissue. Some can be designed with an anterior bow to maintain the position of the anterior segment (Figure 10.2). Hawley retainers are particularly advantageous in mixed dentition, as regular adjustments can be made to the acrylic to accommodate for the eruption of the permanent dentition and to guide the eruption to a degree. It is extremely important that the design of the appliance provides sufficient retention, stability and comfort. Patient motivation and compliance will reduce if the appliance causes discomfort or iatrogenic damage to the soft and hard tissues.

### Vacuum-Formed Retainers

Another popular removable retainer commonly prescribed by orthodontists is the vacuum-formed retainer (Figure 10.3). These are thin thermoplastic materials made over accurate models of teeth following treatment and issued shortly after removal of

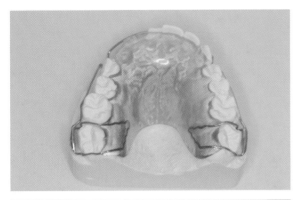

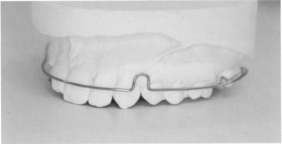

Figure 10.2  Hawley retainer with a labial bow.

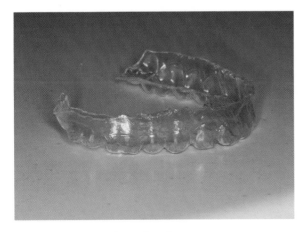

Figure 10.3  Vacuum-formed retainer.

braces. Patients are advised to keep these retainers safe (particularly away from pets) and clean with cold water and tooth brush. Hot water can distort the material. A combined approach of removable and fixed retainers is regularly used. Some can issue vacuum formed retainers to be worn over the bonded retainers to help stabilise the fixed retainers in place for a longer period of time.

## Reference

Mitchell, L. *An Introduction to Orthodontics*. 3rd ed. Oxford: Oxford University Press; 2007.

## Further Reading

Bishara, S. E. *Textbook of Orthodontics*. Philadelphia, PA: W.B. Saunders; 2001.
Burstone, C. J., Marcotte, M. E. *Problem Solving in Orthodontics: Goal-Oriented Treatment Strategies*. Hanover Park, IL: Quintessence; 2000.
Foster, T. D. *A Textbook of Orthodontics*. 3rd ed. Oxford: Blackwell Scientific; 1990.
McDonald, F., Ireland, A. J. *Diagnosis of the Orthodontic Patient*. Oxford: Oxford University Press; 1998.
Nanda, R., Burstone, C. J. (eds). *Retention and Stability in Orthodontics*. Philadelphia, PA: W. B. Saunders; 1993.

## Self-Evaluation

1 What is relapse?
   **A** Teeth showing signs of the initial malocclusion.
   **B** Loss of orthodontic correction.
   **C** Lack of periodontal ligament and gingival fibre adaptation to the orthodontic changes.
   **D** All of the above (a–c).

2 What is retention?
   **A** Prevention of tooth movement during growth.
   **B** Prevention of tooth movement before removal of orthodontic appliances.
   **C** Prevention of tooth movement after removal of orthodontic appliances.
   **D** All of the above (a–c).

3 Which of the following is NOT a removable retainer?
   **A** Twin block.
   **B** Hawley retainer.
   **C** Thermostat vacuum form plastic.
   **D** Multistranded wire on the palatal and lingual surfaces.

4 Upon completion of a course of a functional appliance therapy, reducing appliance wear to nightly wear will provide adequate retention.
   **A** True.
   **B** False.

5 Removable retainers must be active to induce some tooth movement after removal of orthodontic appliances.
   **A** True.
   **B** False.

6  Why is retention necessary?
   **A**  To allow reorganisation of periodontal ligaments and gingival fibres.
   **B**  Neuromuscular adaptations.
   **C**  To allow maturation of osteoid.
   **D**  All of the above (a–c).

7  Which of the following will mostly benefit from permanent retention?
   **A**  Patients with diabetes.
   **B**  Patients with gingivitis.
   **C**  Patients with periodontitis.
   **D**  Patients with cardiovascular diseases.

8  Fixed retainers are micromechanically bonded to enamel for better retention.
   **A**  True.
   **B**  False.

9  Overcorrection is usually recommended to prevent relapse.
   **A**  True.
   **B**  False.

10  For how long after treatment is retention critical?
    **A**  First month.
    **B**  3 months.
    **C**  6 months.
    **D**  12 months.

# 11

# Adult Orthodontics

Over the years, it has become more popular among adults to seek orthodontic treatment for several reasons, such as smile aesthetics, better management of some periodontal conditions and creating space for replacement of missing teeth. Adult orthodontic treatment may be simple or complex depending on the particular problem. Generally, a team of practitioners works together throughout the treatment so the adult can benefit from their orthodontic treatment with minimal impediments and to optimise the outcome.

Periodontists monitor the periodontal condition of the patient and an assessment of the periodontal health status is essential prior to commencement of any orthodontic treatment. Poor periodontal conditions are managed first and stabilised before any orthodontic treatment begins. As part of the treatment, patients might require restorative work such as replacement of missing teeth, general dental management or some cosmetic restorative work to enhance the aesthetics of their smile. Caries, root canals and restorations are managed by dentists prior to orthodontic treatment, as improved oral health is indicated before any orthodontic appliances are fitted. Orthodontic treatment alone may not suffice for some adult patients and orthognathic surgery may be indicated since growth has ceased. In these cases, orthodontists work closely with oral maxillofacial surgeons to achieve the desired results and to address chief complaints.

## Orthognathic Surgery

The details of orthognathic surgery are not discussed in depth in this chapter, as this is outside the scope of this textbook. Some of the common jaw surgeries are briefly identified to advance your awareness as oral health therapists, dental hygienists and dental therapists in this area.

Orthognathic surgery is the term given to oral maxillofacial surgery planned in combination with orthodontic treatment to correct skeletal deformities associated with soft tissue, dento-osseous syndrome and musculoskeletal anomalies. This approach is usually indicated if growth modification or camouflage treatment will not be sufficient to correct the orthodontic problem. The therapeutic objective for this approach is to treat severe skeletal discrepancies that cannot solely be treated with orthodontics, to reduce treatment time and aid in enhancing treatment stability. However, surgery does not replace orthodontic treatment but is rather used in combination with orthodontic treatment.

*Orthodontics for Dental Hygienists and Dental Therapists*, First Edition. Tina Raked.
© 2018 John Wiley & Sons Ltd. Published 2018 by John Wiley & Sons Ltd.
Companion website: www.wiley.com/go/raked/orthodontics_dental_hygienists

Orthognathic surgery is usually delayed until the patient has reached skeletal maturity to eliminate the risk of relapse from continuous growth. An exception to this is for patients suffering from morphological disorders or craniofacial anomalies, such as cleft lip and palate, which require early surgical intervention. Correction of severe skeletal discrepancies not only improves the facial profile but also enhances the psychosocial wellbeing, the aesthetics and function of the occlusion, and improves speech and masticatory functions. Diagnosis and management of cases with orthognathic surgery involves a team of dental practitioners led by an oral maxillofacial surgeon and an orthodontist. The craniomaxillofacial structure is complex, so extensive examination and planning are indicated. Apart from a thorough orthodontic examination, a detailed facial assessment, radiographic evaluation, extra- and intraoral examinations are needed by the surgeon for planning the surgical procedures. To achieve the desired facial appearance in some cases, the patient might require other facial surgical corrections, such as rhinoplasty. The details of treatment and procedures should be discussed with the patient carefully so they are given the opportunity to make an informed decision. In some practices, computer programs can provide patient images to create visual predictions for the various changes that will occur in their facial profile and appearance for their treatment options.

Once the gathered data have been studied carefully by the team of specialists, a diagnosis is made for skeletal or temporomandibular joint dysfunction, musculature defects, dental and occlusal abnormalities. The skeletal diagnosis made includes both jaws in all planes of space (vertical, sagittal and transverse), the direction of the problem and whether it is an excess or deficiency of each jaw. A problem may be detected in one arch or both dental arches. Generally, surgery is indicated in patients with skeletal maturity. Patients suffering from deficiencies most benefit from early treatment, while patients with defects associated with protrusion of the jaws achieve better results with delayed surgical correction. Continuous growth has minimal effect on patients with jaw deficiencies, although there is a higher risk of relapse associated with excess or protrusive jaws treated too early.

A successful orthognathic treatment includes the following outcomes:

- functional and aesthetic occlusion
- absence of temporomandibular joint dysfunction
- preserved periodontal health
- no musculofascial pain
- maintain or increased airway
- maintain facial balance
- chief complaint addressed.

As with all surgical procedures, orthognathic surgery can also have complications associated with it. Every individual undergoing the surgery will experience different post-operational adverse effects. Some of the common post-surgical complications are as follows:

- numbness and tingling in the jaws
- swelling
- bruising
- nasal congestion

- discomfort during sleep
- xerostomia (dry mouth)
- dry lips.

The choice of surgery varies depending on which jaw is diagnosed with the anomaly by the team of specialists. Certain orthodontic goals can be achieved before surgery and some final adjustments are necessary after surgery. Generally, the presurgical orthodontic intention is removal of dental compensations. This is the opposite of treating patients with extractions. If a patient is treated with extractions, the objective is to enhance and use the dentoalveolar compensations to camouflage the occlusal discrepancies. For this critical reason, it is extremely important that the team of practitioners and the patient follow a well-understood treatment plan, as opposite approaches are used to correct the problem. Hence, it will become complicated if decisions are changed mid-treatment. Once the necessary changes are made and the patient has been orthodontically prepared, the surgical correction takes place under general anaesthesia. The final adjustments and orthodontic corrections are made post-surgery in subsequent visits to achieve the desired functional and aesthetic results.

### Presurgery Orthodontic Goals

Generally, dental compensations are removed prior to surgery and alignments are corrected. Dental compensations are dentoalveolar changes that disguise the skeletal discrepancies. For example, tipping back of the lower incisors in a skeletal class III patient camouflages the abnormal jaw position. The main objective of eliminating dentoalveolar compensations is to create sufficient horizontal space between the upper and lower incisors to allow better shift of the jaws and to improve the inter incisal relationship, which will greatly improve the facial profile of the patient. Other presurgical goals are to:

- correct alignment
- relieve crowding
- confirm arch form compatibility
- create space for osteotomy (surgical sectioning of the bone)
- level and flatten the curve of Spee
- level the curve of Wilson

### Post-surgery Orthodontic Goals

Post-surgery goals include detailing the occlusion and root paralleling. Some of the common postoperative instructions that patients need to be made aware of include:

- a liquid diet for two to four weeks
- modified diet up to six weeks
- can return to work within two weeks
- no contact sports for up to 12 weeks
- might require corticosteroids to reduce swelling
- depending on the type of surgery, some patients may require elastic wear as instructed by the orthodontist for better patient comfort and guidance of the occlusion
- some patients may require physiotherapy to regain full function.

## Maxillary Surgical Procedures

### Le Forte Osteotomy

Le Forte osteotomy is a surgical procedure to correct maxillary abnormalities and to redirect the maxilla in the desired position downwards, forwards or backwards. Depending on the plane in which the osteotomy takes place, this surgical technique is categorised in three groups of Le Fort I, Le Forte II and Le Forte III (Figure 11.1). Le Forte I is commonly used in vertical maxillary excess. A gummy smile is one of the common clinical signs of a vertical maxillary excess. Le Fort I is also commonly used for correction of open bite. The maxilla is levelled and moved posteriorly and upwards providing highly stable outcomes. Relapse is associated with downward movement of the maxilla as it also requires bone grafting. The soft tissue dissection to access the maxilla is across the upper labial vestibular region, superior to the molars regions and inferior to the anterior nasal spine. The bony cut takes place from the edge of the anterior nasal floor known as the pyriform rim and along the lateral surfaces of the maxilla where the zygomatic arch meets the maxilla. This bony cut extends to the pterygoid plate region. The nasal floor is elevated and the nasal septum is separated from the maxilla with surgical instruments. The lateral borders of the nose are also separated with a bony incision. Care is taken to preserve the greater palatine neurovascular bundle as the maxilla is separated and stabilised.

The osteotomy takes place on several landmarks to mobilise the maxilla and articulate it in the desired position. Plates and screws are used to secure the new position as articulated against the mandible. Inter maxillary fixation is removed post-surgery and, to enhance the stability of the results, elastic wear as instructed by the orthodontist is critical. In Le Forte II and Le Forte III, larger areas are mobilised. Le Forte II osteotomy involves the inferior orbital rim and the nasal bridge. Le Forte III is a transverse incision in the bone across the nasal bridge and the orbit extending down the zygomatic arch.

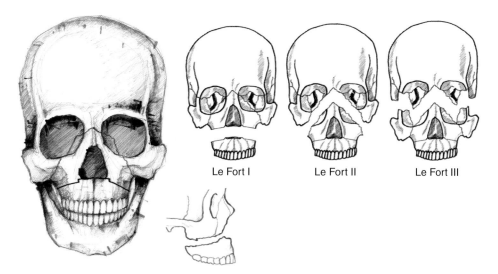

Le Fort I          Le Fort II          Le Fort III

Figure 11.1 Le Forte osteotomy.

One of the risks associated with this surgery is temporary altered sensation in the maxillary region, upper lip and nose.

### Surgically Assisted Rapid Palatal Expansion

In severe maxillary transverse discrepancies, patients are treated with surgically assisted rapid palatal expansion also known as surgically assisted maxillary expansion. This surgical procedure is a type of distraction osteogenesis, which is a surgical procedure that results in extending the length of a bone. It is indicated in patients who have reached skeletal maturity and are diagnosed with a severe narrow maxilla resulting in cross bites and requiring significant maxillary expansion (Figures 11.2 and 11.3).

Treating children and young adolescents with an orthopaedic appliance such as a maxillary expander will suffice for correction of a narrow maxilla. However, surgical assistance for adults allows the split of the palatine suture and enhances the stability of the treatment. This surgical technique is a combination of a rapid maxillary expander with a modified Le Forte I osteotomy. The expander is fitted before the surgery. The bone incision is from the first molar region towards the midline close to the palatine suture bilaterally. Another cut in the bone is made along the lateral surfaces of the maxilla and over the anterior nasal spine superior to the central incisor apices. The palatal suture is gently tapped open by placing a chisel into the vertical cut and mobilising the posterior segments. The appliance is activated to stabilise the split of the maxillary suture. The expansion of the plate post-surgery occurs at a rate decided by the surgeon and the orthodontist. There can be several variations and modifications made to this surgical technique as decided by the team of specialists. It is critical to advise the patient that a significant midline diastema will occur following surgery.

## Mandibular Surgical Procedures

### Bilateral Sagittal Split Osteotomy

Bilateral sagittal split osteotomy is a surgical technique that can be used to advance or retrude the mandible. The osteotomy takes place on a sagittal dimension of the mandibular body and ramus. The patient is treated under general anaesthesia and the soft-tissue incision is made intraorally, extending from the first molar region and along to the coronoid process to expose the underlying bone. The first osteotomy is made horizontally, reaching about two-thirds of the ramus from the anterior border of the mandible to the posterior border of the mandible. This cut extends into the cancellous bone located inferiorly to the coronoid notch and superior to the inferior alveolar foramen.

The second osteotomy extends sagittally from the tip of the first bony cut down the ramus of the mandible. This sectioning is about one millimetre medial to the external oblique line (Figure 11.4). The objective is to gain three fragments by splitting the mandible: one fragment is the anterior portion containing the teeth and two posterior fragments bearing the mandibular condyle. The bone incisions are carefully made, preserving the inferior alveolar nerve.

The mandible is split after the incisions are made in the ramus and is widened to allow free movement of the coronoid process and the condyle. Once the split in the ramus is

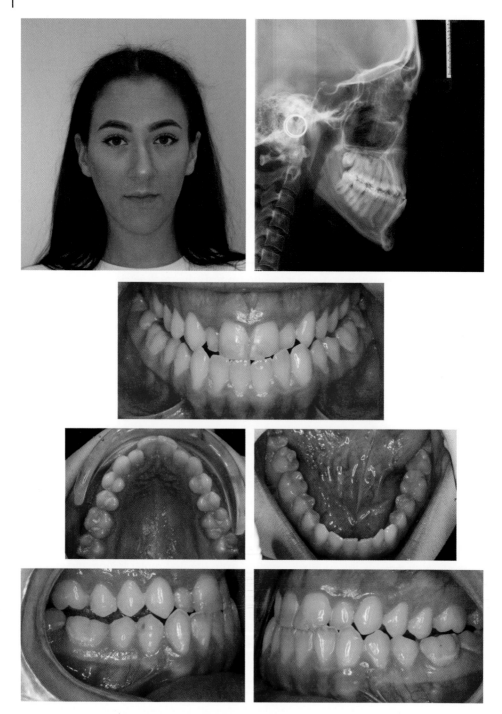

**Figure 11.2** Surgically assisted rapid palatal expansion case prior to surgery. *Source*: Case by Dr Shimanto Purkayastha and Dr Peter Tsakiris.

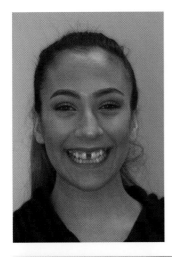
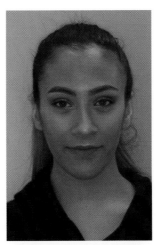
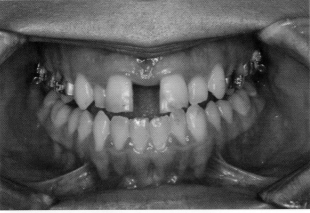
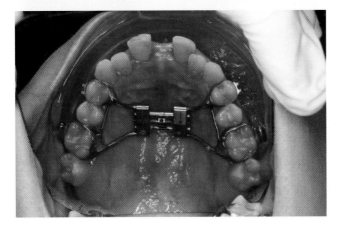

**Figure 11.3** Development of a large median diastema gained from surgically assisted rapid palatal expansion.

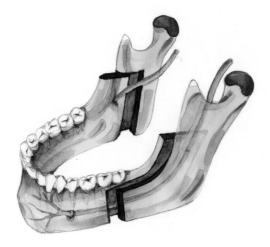

Figure 11.4 Bilateral split osteotomy.

achieved bilaterally, intermaxillary fixation is achieved by ligating upper and lower arches together with wires to position the mandible forwards or backwards, to attain the desired occlusion. Rigid fixation of the mandible secures the jaw in the new position with plates and 2-mm positional screws that allows natural bone growth to take place between the pieces. The patient is usually discharged within 24 hours in the absence of complications.

Follow-up appointments are scheduled with the surgeon to monitor healing. Regular orthodontic visits are necessary to achieve the post-surgical finishing. To guide the occlusion, patient will require elastic wear as instructed by the orthodontist. Upon completion of the orthodontic treatment, the patient will require regular review appointments with the orthodontist and the surgeon to check the retention and stability of the treatment outcome. The risks associated with this procedure are sensory complications due to exposure of the inferior alveolar neurovascular canal. The patients can experience numbness in the area following the surgery for several months. Moving the mandible forward causes stretching of the suprahyoid muscle complex. Advancement of the lower jaw more than seven millimetres with this procedure has been associated with a degree of relapse.

### Genioplasty

The surgical technique used to correct abnormalities in the chin is termed genioplasty. A soft-tissue incision in the anterior mandibular vestibular region extending to the canine region allows access to the chin. This procedure is carried out with care to protect and preserve the nerves in the area. This procedure aids in correcting:

- symphysis deformities
- excessive prominence of the chin
- vertical defects in the chin
- flat or retrusive chin.

With this surgical technique, the chin can be moved forwards or backwards, or it may be tilted, narrowed or widened. To gain this correction, a horizontal bony cut is made in the chin and redirected in the desired position (Figure 11.5). The length of the chin

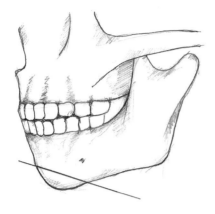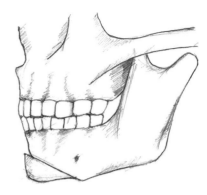

Figure 11.5 Genioplasty.

can be extended if moved forwards or shortened with osteotomy (removal of bone). To reduce or increase the width of the chin, a division is made in the centre. The stability of the treatment is usually gained with plates and screws.

## Bimaxillary Osteotomy

In some patients, both upper and lower arches will present with deformities. The team of specialists decides on bimaxillary osteotomy and correct both arches. Surgeons will keep one jaw stabilised at all times during the surgery to achieve the desired occlusion. The sequence in which the bony cuts take place is rearranged as decided by the surgeon. For example, the maxillary osteotomy can be made and the upper arch positioned and rotated as needed without splitting the mandible. After correction of the upper jaw, the position of the mandible is decided accordingly.

## Post-Condylar Cartilage Graft

The mandible can be advanced with post-condylar cartilage grafting in some patients with a retrusive mandible.

### Case Study

An example of an orthognathic treatment is shown in the case presented in Figures 11.6, 11.7 and 11.8. The patient presented with the following:

- concave profile
- brachyfacial type
- skeletal class III due to a retrusive maxilla presenting with a mid-face retrognathism
- angle class III malocclusion
- initially, cephalometric findings indicated proclined maxillary anterior teeth, which are compensated as a result of this class III skeletal base
- an asymmetric occlusion with the maxillary dental midline coinciding with the facial midline

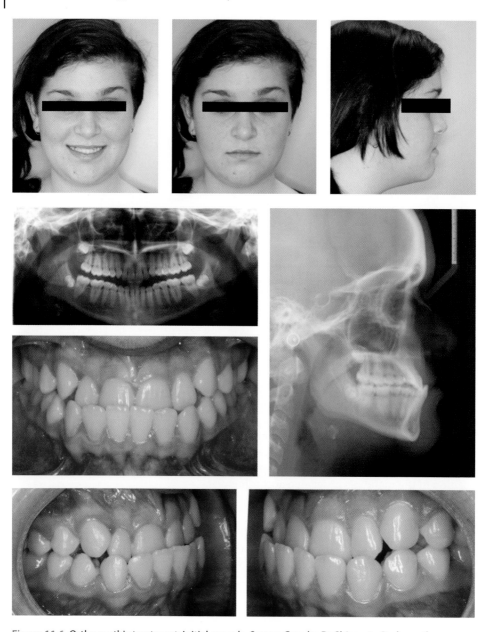

Figure 11.6 Orthognathic treatment; initial records. *Source*: Case by Dr Shimanto Purkayastha.

The treatment objectives were to:

- improve the facial profile
- improve the skeletal base relationship
- correct under bite
- relieve crowding
- align and level the dental arches

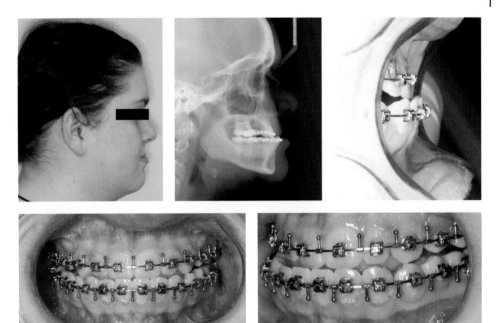

Figure 11.7 Orthognathic treatment; pre-surgical photographs. As a result of an asymmetric occlusion, after decompensation, the patient presented with an asymmetric class III malocclusion, which was addressed at the time of surgery with a mandibular osteotomy.

- coordinate the dental arch forms
- align and coordinate the midlines
- establish a class I molar relationship
- establish a class I canine relationship
- reduce or eliminate any temporomandibular joint pain or discomfort
- reduce or eliminate any psychosocial issues regarding teeth and smile
- produce stable treatment results.

Treatment was in several stages. Upper and lower fixed appliances were placed using a self-ligating 0.022-inch preadjusted edgewise prescription with selective torques to decompensate the teeth before the surgery. The upper first premolars were extracted under general anaesthesia at the same time that the third molars were removed. A transpalatal arch was placed for anchorage. Subsequent orthognathic surgery involved Le Forte 1 and mandibular osteotomies. Retention involved a fixed lingual retainer in the upper and lower arches with a removable maxillary retainer in the upper arch.

## Clear Aligners

Over the years, there has been a paradigm shift in treating adults and adolescents with the introduction of clear aligner therapy as an alternative to braces. One of the most popular and widely used aligner technologies is Invisalign®, which was introduced in 1997 and is the focus of this chapter. The suitability of the patient for this type of therapy is best diagnosed by an orthodontist.

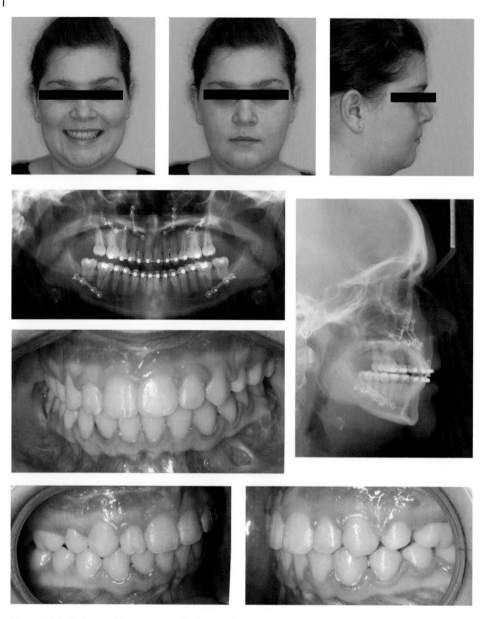

**Figure 11.8** Orthognathic treatment; final records. *Source*: Courtesy of Dr Shimanto Purkayastha.

Mild to moderate discrepancies can be treated with this innovative technology. The assessment and diagnostic processes do not differ from any other orthodontic treatment. Once an informed consent is gained from the patient, a three-dimensional digital model is made and the aligners are manufactured in the Invisalign laboratories. Polyvinyl siloxane impressions or a digital scan of the teeth are sent to specified dental laboratories. The digital models of the teeth are used by technicians to create a treatment plan and to design a series of tooth movements with ClinCheck, a software program developed by the company. The orthodontist works closely with the technicians to provide advice on the goals of treatment and supervise the desired outcomes prior to manufacturing of the aligners.

The aligners are modelled with computer-aided design and manufacturing (CAD-CAM). The CAD data are used to fabricate a three-dimensional model using stereolithography, which is a type of three-dimensional printing using various techniques known as rapid technology prototyping. The aligners are composed of an elastic thermoplastic material to create force against the tooth and the attachments that are bonded on to the teeth to allow movement. Teeth will move as directed by a series of aligners for a better fit.

Together with the set of manufactured aligners, a template aligner will be processed for bonding the attachments to the teeth. If additional tooth movements are needed during treatment with additional attachments, another template is included in the series prior to fitting the aligner with extra attachments. To gain space for better tooth movement interproximal enamel reduction is planned by the orthodontist at various stages of treatment. Interproximal enamel reduction or slenderising is removal of interproximal enamel to create the space necessary. This is not confined to aligner technology and may also be incorporated as part of fixed appliance therapy. A Bolton's analysis is a good indicator as to how much reduction is necessary for the patient. This technique also prevents the formation of black triangles.

Every aligner moves the teeth 0.25–0.33 mm. The objective is to create low continuous forces to achieve proportional root and crown movement and to prevent hyalinisation and root resorption. Each aligner is worn for about one to two weeks or as instructed by the orthodontist, usually for 20–22 hours a day. Only a few aligners are given to the patient, as instructed by the orthodontist. Some specialists may prefer more frequent check-ups to track the treatment progress closely, so they only issue a few aligners at every appointment and organise frequent return visits. Some orthodontists prefer longer tracking of the treatment, thus provide the patient with more aligners and organising the visits with longer intervals.

### Attachments

A series of attachments of various shapes are designed on the digital model on specific teeth that require movement. Attachments are also a great source of anchorage. Various shapes are responsible for different tooth movements. Examples of these specific movements with various attachments are:

- rectangular:
  A bevelled horizontal rectangular attachment will result in extrusion. Vertical rectangles on premolars will result in rotation. This causes anterior intrusion when bonded bilaterally and on the first premolar in each quadrant. Vertical rectangles aid in uprighting the root axis.
- ellipsoidal:
  A horizontal ellipsoidal will result in extrusion. Vertical ellipsoidal attachments provide aligner retention.
- tear drop:
  On canines, this will result in rotation.

The bonded attachments on the teeth are typically smaller than the aligners. Optimised attachments are composed of active and passive surfaces that engage with the aligner and initiate the designated movement based on the shape. The passive surfaces acts as anchorage. Power ridges provide lingual root torque and pressure points on the aligner that aids root movement control in buccal and lingual movements. Power ridges and attachments are not used concomitantly on the same tooth. The objective of optimised attachments is to change the shape of the tooth to activate the aligners once engaged on to the active surfaces resulting in a mechanical interference creating low continuous forces.

To facilitate elastic wear, aligners can be designed with precision cuts for elastic hooks and buttons around canines, premolars and molars (Figures 11.9 and 11.10).

### Bonding Attachments

The steps involved in bonding Invisalign attachments are as follows (Figure 11.11):

1) The tooth surface is prepared with pumice and rinsed thoroughly with water to remove debris and plaque. A clean surface enhances bonding.
2) The enamel of the teeth that will have attachments bonded can be microetched with aluminium oxide to enhance bonding.

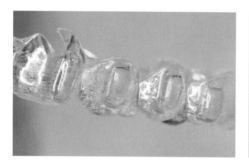 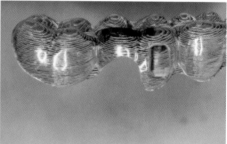

**Figure 11.9** Aligners precision cut for elastic wear. The cut-out on the molar region is to allow bonding of buttons for elastic wear.

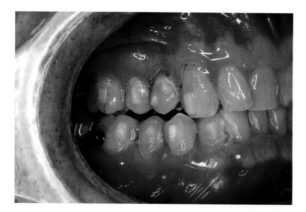

**Figure 11.10** Attachments bonded to teeth with a button on the lower first molars for class II elastic wear from the lower molars to the precision cut on the upper canines on the aligner.

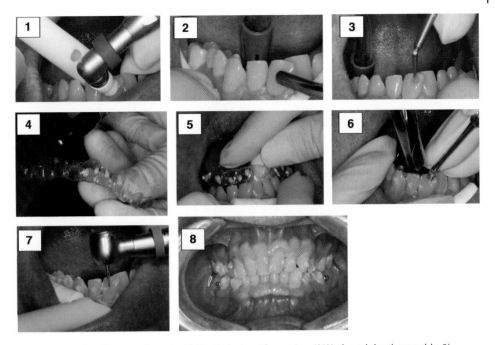

Figure 11.11 Bonding attachments: 1) Prophylaxis with pumice. 2) Wash and dry thoroughly. 3) Prepare the enamel surface with self-etching primer lollipop (etch and bond can be used instead of the lollipop). 4) Load the template aligner with composite. 5) Fit the template aligner on the teeth. 6) Gently press attachments with a band pusher and set the composite. 7) Remove the aligner and the excess composite. 8) Check that all the attachments are bonded on the teeth.

3) A dry working field and good control of saliva is critical for better bonding strength. Cotton rolls, cheek and tongue retractors are used for saliva control.

4) A self-etching primer is used to prepare the teeth.

5) The attachment template is filled with composite and placed over the teeth. Prior to setting the composite, a firm pressure is exerted against the attachments with a band pusher.

6) Once the composite is set, the template is removed and the excess is polished with a carbide bur.

7) Care must be given not to damage the edges of the attachment and the enamel surface. The edges of the attachments are the active sites and the shape must be maintained. Floss the contacts to ensure adhesives are removed interproximally.

### Interproximal Enamel Reduction

If interproximal enamel reduction is indicated, the procedure is as follows:

1) A diamond-coated disc or strip can be used to remove a thin layer of enamel interproximally.

2) This is an abrasive technique and can increase the risk of caries if bacteria are collected in the area on the rough surfaces. Slenderising is therefore recommended with fluoridated prophylaxis to create a smoother surface (Alexander, 2008).

3) The treatment plan provides a guide for the amount and site of interproximal enamel reduction. The wheel is gently inserted in the contact point to remove the desired amount of enamel.
4) Protection of the lip and tongue is critical for this procedure.
5) To check the space created, interproximal enamel reduction keys (Figure 11.12) are placed in the contact points to provide a reading of space gained interproximally.

Interproximal enamel reduction can be achieved in many ways. One example is a diamond-coated disc with a handpiece (Figure 11.13). Care must be given when using this technique as it rapidly removes enamel. Another example is the orthodontic interproximal enamel reduction strip (Figure 11.14).

### Patient Care Instructions for Clear Aligners

The aligners must be worn at all times and removed before eating or drinking, with an exception to drinking cold water. If the aligners are worn during drinking wine or coffee, it will accumulate in the aligners for a prolonged period of time and will

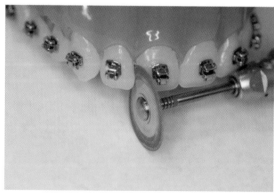

Figure 11.12 Interproximal reduction keys to measure the amount of interproximal reduction achieved.

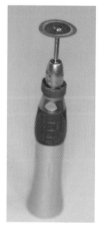
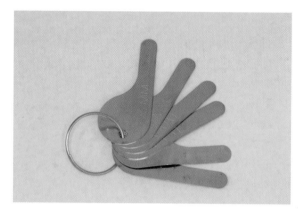

Figure 11.13 A diamond coated disc with a straight handpiece used for interproximal reduction.

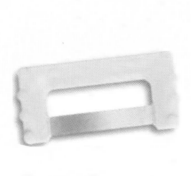

Figure 11.14 Orthodontic interproximal reduction strip.

greatly increase the risk of caries and enamel wear due to acid attacks. The aligners are safe to be worn during sleep and sports. They should always be handled with clean hands.

One aligner should be worn at a time: do not try to place both upper and lower aligners in at the same time. They are best cleaned with cold water and a toothbrush. A Minimal amount of toothpaste must be used to prevent wear of the aligners over time. They should not be cleaned with denture cleansers, as these will damage the aligner surfaces, making them more visible as they become dulled.

Once removed from the mouth, the aligners must be kept in the case to prevent loss or damage to the aligners. If the treatment plan involves the use of elastics, the patient must be advised on the pattern and duration of elastic wear, as instructed by the orthodontist.

In some cases, patients might not be eligible to continue their course of aligners, as a change in the initial treatment plan may be indicated, thus requiring a mid-course correction. Upon completion of a course of aligners, orthodontists may decide that further correction is needed requiring a refinement phase with additional aligners to reach the treatment objectives. The attachments are removed and further records, impressions or scans are gathered for the orthodontist to make further corrections to the occlusion and order another set of aligners that will produce the final ideal results. The patient is advised to wear the last aligner nightly to retain the teeth in position until the new aligners arrive.

### Removing Attachments

To remove the attachments, the following steps are followed:

1) The enamel surface is dried to distinguish the layer of composite and enamel better.
2) A carbide bur is used to remove the composite attachments.
3) Use of an ultrasonic scaler is also helpful to remove any residual composite once the attachments are polished with a carbide bur.

An example of Invisalign treatment is presented in Figures 11.15 to 11.16. The patient presented with the following:

- straight profile
- mesofacial skeletal base
- 6-mm overjet
- traumatic overbite
- lower anterior crowding
- class II division 1
- class II canine relationship
- class I molar relationship.

The skeletal base exhibited a class II profile with a retrusive mandible at an increased vertical dimension. The main concern of the patient was lower anterior crowding, and the option of surgical correction of the underlying skeletal discrepancy was declined. The chosen treatment option was a non-extraction alignment only. This was achieved with sequential plastic aligners to relieve the anterior crowding. The aligners were used with class II elastic wear to address the class II dental relationship.

# Lingual Braces

Adults and teenagers seek aesthetic options for orthodontic treatment because of the perceived embarrassment of labial braces. Lingual brackets were introduced in the 1970s by Dr Cravern Kurz. Early designs impeded speech, irritated the tongue, impinged on the gingival margin and interfered with occlusion. The original brackets were direct bonded, compromising the accuracy of bracket placement leading to unpredictable alignments.

Since the introduction of lingual braces, there have been several systems and designs introduced in lingual orthodontics to improve the efficiency, quality and comfort of the treatment. Some improvements include smooth edges to reduce irritation to the tongue; a lower profile and seating of the brackets about 1–2 mm from the gingival margin to prevent impingement and aids in cleaning the brackets. A bite plane effect was incorporated in the design of the bracket to improve occlusal interference an indirect bonding technique greatly enhanced the accuracy of bracket placement, therefore improving the tip and torque. The brackets were redesigned with ball hooks that are not too close to the gingival margin, for better ligation of modules. The mesial aperture of molar tubes was widened to allow better wire insertion. Self-ligating lingual brackets have also been developed.

Lingual brackets do have some disadvantages yet they also have great advantages over labial brackets. Irritation to the tongue and difficulty in speech improves within two to three weeks after placement of brackets. Apart from the apparent aesthetic appeal, lingual brackets present with reduced white spot lesions and a lower caries risk. The lingual surfaces are less prone to decay and caries in comparison to buccal surfaces. The brackets are customised and contoured closely to the morphology of the lingual surfaces and, in cases of good cementation, most of the enamel in the lingual area is sealed (Van der Veen et al., 2010). Examples of some of the lingual systems used include Incognito™, Win and In-Ovation® Lingual.

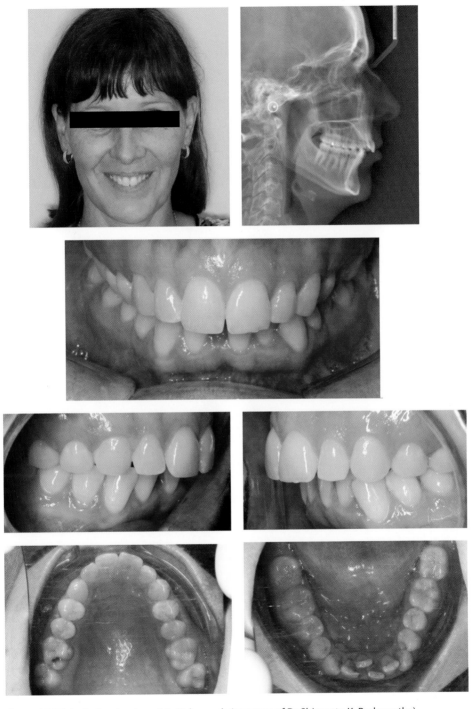

Figure 11.15 Invisalign treatment; initial records (courtesy of Dr Shimanto K. Purkayastha).

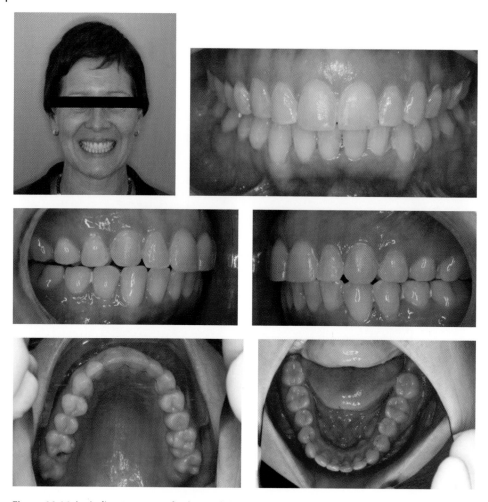

Figure 11.16 Invisalign treatment; final records (courtesy of Dr Shimanto K. Purkayastha).

### Lingual Orthodontic Mechanics

The biomechanics of lingual braces differ from labial braces. Lighter forces are created with a shorter interbracket distance and lower arch circumference. The lingual brackets are positioned palatal and closer to the centre of resistance of the tooth due to the morphology of the lingual surfaces. Lingual braces allow passive extrusive forces on the posterior teeth and active intrusive forces on the anterior teeth to facilitate deep bite correction by maintaining the maxillomandibular relationship. Lingual braces have shown to aid in expansion of the maxillary arch. It is not fully understood how this expansive effect is achieved. The theories used to explain this effect are the interbracket width, thickness of the bracket and direction of force from inside the arch towards the outside.

Lingual appliances have unique mechanical characteristics that allow more effective results to be achieved in four areas in comparison with labial appliances (Romano, 2011):

1) Intrusion of anterior teeth.
2) Maxillary arch expansion.

3) Distalisation of maxillary molars.
4) Combining mandibular repositioning therapy with orthodontic movement.

### Positioning the Lingual Bracket

Several systems have been introduced to enhance treatment efficacy by increasing the accuracy of bonding lingual brackets. High-quality polyvinyl siloxane impressions or digital scans of the teeth are used to send to laboratories with specific diagnostic instructions by orthodontists. The treatment goals and anticipated tooth movements are communicated between the specialists and laboratory technicians to produce accurate and desirable outcomes. Customised bracket positions on the lingual surfaces and a series of arch wires to reach the treatment objectives are manufactured using various techniques and programs. Some of the systems developed are:

- the customised lingual appliance set-up service (CLASS) system
- the torque angulation reference guide (TARG)
- the bonding with equal specific thickness (BEST) system
- the Hiro system
- the Slot Machine
- the mushroom bracket positioner
- the lingual bracket Jig
- transfer Optimised positioning
- CAD/CAM system.

### Bonding

Lingual brackets are best bonded indirectly. The brackets are manufactured in laboratories with transfer trays, as accurate direct bonding of the brackets to lingual surfaces may be extremely difficult with limited access and field of vision. Orthodontists may have a specific preferred method in bonding lingual brackets and there are various systems used by different specialists. A brief summary of indirect bonding lingual brackets is as follows:

1) Achieve sufficient isolation using cheek and tongue retractors to maintain a dry working field.
2) Prophylaxis to remove debris and plaque from the lingual surfaces.
3) Microetch the lingual surfaces to enhance bonding strength and prevent bonding failures.
4) Etch using orthophosphoric acid 37% for 15–30 seconds.
5) Wash and dry thoroughly and try the bonding trays to ensure the brackets are seated nicely against the lingual surfaces prior to cementation.
6) Once the fit of the tray is approved, dry the brackets thoroughly and apply adhesive to the base.
7) Prepare the enamel surface with a primer as instructed by the specialist.
8) Gently seat the tray and press a firm pressure on the brackets and set the adhesive.
9) Remove the tray and any excess adhesives surrounding the brackets, particularly from the gingival margins.
10) Before insertion of the wire, check every bracket to ensure that the bonding is strong.

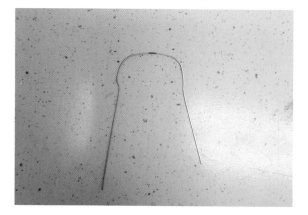

Figure 11.17 Customised lingual arch wire. *Source*: Nour Eldin Tarraf.

### Lingual Arch Wires

Lingual arch wires differ from labial arch wires and are 'mushroom' shaped due to the lingual arch form. The lingual wires are preformed and can be composed of either nickel titanium, stainless steel or beta-titanium. They are designed to be used at various stages of treatment as instructed by the orthodontist. Typically, a shape memory alloy is used in the initial stages to achieve rapid alignment and initial levelling (Figure 11.17).

### Patients with Lingual Braces

Initially, lingual braces were introduced as an aesthetic option for orthodontic treatment in adults. However, children in late mixed dentition may also be suitable candidates for this type of treatment. Orthodontists may find many patients who are not suitable for such a treatment, depending on the presenting orthodontic problem. Other factors that influence the decision of the specialist on offering lingual orthodontics to patients include:

- patient motivation
- oral hygiene
- aesthetics and patient self-image
- periodontal health.

### Lingual Braces Case Study

Lingual braces can be used in patients requiring orthognathic surgery; however, some labial braces will be bonded prior to surgery to aid rigid fixation. An example of treating class II division 2 with lingual braces is seen in Figures 11.18–11.21. The patient presented with the following:

- convex profile with mandibular retrusion
- low smile line
- class II division 2 on a class II skeletal base
- 100% deep bite
- square upper arch with retroclined upper central incisors
- scissor bite on the upper right first premolar
- square lower arch
- coincident upper and lower midlines.

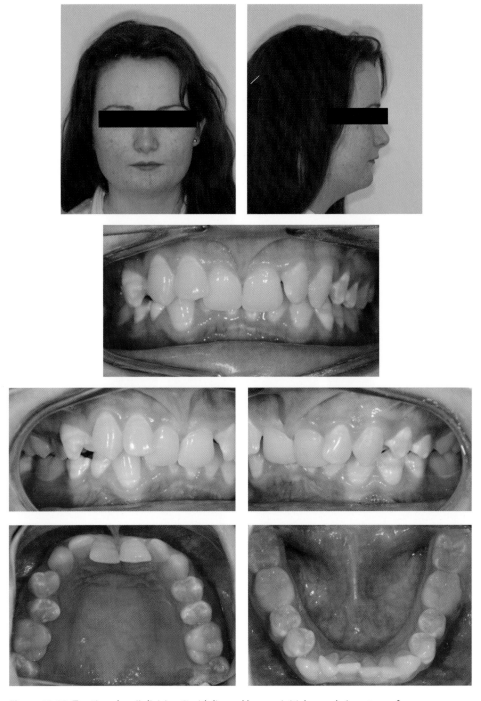

Figure 11.18 Treating class II division 2 with lingual braces; initial records (courtesy of Dr Nour Eldin Tarraf).

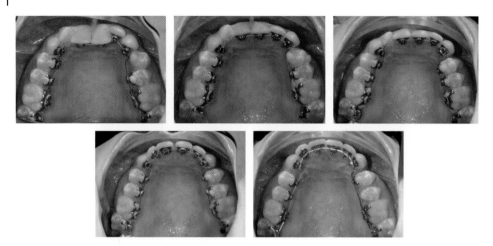

Figure 11.19 Expansion of the upper arch is evident over time as the anterior maxillary teeth are proclined.

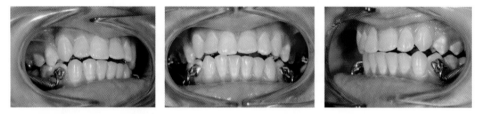

Figure 11.20 A Forsus appliance used to posture the mandible forwards and address the skeletal class II after correction of the deep bite and proclination of the upper incisors has been achieved.

The patient was treated with upper and lower fixed lingual braces and a fixed functional appliance (Forsus) to address the skeletal discrepancy.

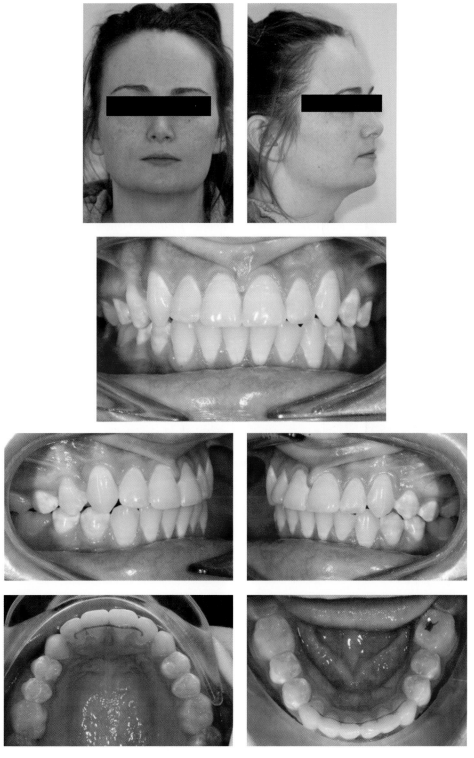

Figure 11.21 Treating class II division 2 with lingual braces; final records (courtesy of Dr Nour Eldin Tarraf).

## References

Alexander, R. G. *The 20 Principles of the Alexander Discipline*. Hanover Park IL: Quintessence; 2008.

Romano, R. *Lingual and Esthetic Orthodontics*. Hanover Park, IL: Quintessence; 2011.

Van der Veen, M. H., Attin, R., Schweska-Polly, R., et al. Caries outcomes after with fixed appliances: do lingual brackets make a difference? *Eur J Oral Sci*, 2010; 118: 298–303.

## Further Reading

Bishara, S. E. *Textbook of Orthodontics*. Philadelphia, PA: W.B. Saunders; 2001.

Bouchez, R. *Clinical Success in Invisalign Orthodontic Treatment*. Hanover Park, IL: Quintessence; 2010.

Brand, R. W., Isselhard, D. E. *Anatomy of Orofacial Structures: A comprehensive approach*. 7th ed. St Louis, MO: Elsevier Mosby.

Downs, W. B. Analysis of the dentofacial profile. *Angle Orthod*, 1956; 26(4): 191–212.

Foster, T. D. *A Textbook of Orthodontics*. 3rd ed. Oxford: Blackwell Scientific; 1990.

Goose, D. H., Appleton, J. *Human Dentofacial Growth*. Oxford: Pergamon Press; 1982.

Ling, P. H. Lingual orthodontics: history, misconceptions and clarification. *J Can Dent Assoc*, 2005; 71(2): 99–102.

Mitchell, L. *An Introduction to Orthodontics*. 3rd ed. Oxford: Oxford University Press; 2007.

Mori, Y., Takafumi Susami, Hideto Saijo, et al. Mandibular body osteoctomy for correction of mandibular prognathism: a technical note. *Oral Sci Int*, 2012; 9: 21–25.

Ranly, D. M. (ed.) *A Synopsis of Craniofacial Growth*. Norwalk, CT: Appleton and Lange; 1988.

Thilander, B. Basic mechanisms in craniofacial growth. *Acta Odontol Scand*, 1995; 53(3): 144–151.

Welbury, R. R., Duggal, M. S., Hosey, M. T. *Paediatric Dentistry*. 4th ed. Oxford: Oxford University Press; 2012.

Wiet, G. J. Biavati, M. J., Rocha-Worley, G. Reconstructive surgery for cleft palate treatment and management. *Medscape*, 17 August 2015. Available at http://emedicine.medscape.com/article/878062-treatment (accessed 7 April 2017).

Wiechmann, D. Lingual orthodontics (part 1): laboratory procedure. *J Orofac Orthop*, 1999; 60(5): 371–379.

## Self-Evaluation

1   Dental compensations are removed orthodontically prior to surgery.
    **A**  True.
    **B**  False.

2   Which term is given to the type of orthognathic surgery that extends bone length?
    **A**  Le forte II.
    **B**  Genioplasty.
    **C**  Distraction osteogenesis.
    **D**  Le Forte III.

3 The most stable surgical results are achieved if patient has NOT reached a skeletal maturity.
   **A** True.
   **B** False.

4 Which of the following procedures are a low-level osteotomy?
   **A** Lefort I.
   **B** Lefort II.
   **C** Lefort III.
   **D** Distraction osteogenesis.

5 Which of the following surgical procedures allows retraction of the chin?
   **A** Vertical subsigmoid osteotomy.
   **B** Sagittal split osteotomy
   **C** Genioplasty.
   **D** Body osteotomy.

6 What is the aim of bonding attachments for clear aligner therapy?
   **A** To make tooth movement possible with a series of aligners.
   **B** To achieve specific tooth movements on each tooth.
   **C** To have more control over movement of teeth.
   **D** All of the above (a–c).

7 How many hours must the aligners be worn to achieve effective outcomes?
   **A** 10–12 hours.
   **B** 20–22 hours.
   **C** 6–8 hours.
   **D** 16–18 hours.

8 In which areas have lingual orthodontics shown to be more effective than labial braces?
   **A** Distalisation of maxillary molars.
   **B** Maxillary expansion.
   **C** Intrusion of anterior teeth.
   **D** All of the above.

9 What are power ridges on aligners?
   **A** Delivers force on the tooth for specific movements.
   **B** Allows correction of inclination of teeth.
   **C** Provides a better torque control.
   **D** All of the above (a–c).

10 All areas of the attachments are active.
   **A** True.
   **B** False.

# Self-Evaluation Answers

## Chapter 2

1) b
2) a
3) a
4) b
5) a
6) b
7) d
8) d
9) c
10) c

## Chapter 3

1) d
2) a
3) c
4) e
5) e
6) d
7) c
8) c
9) c
10) c

## Chapter 4

1) a
2) b
3) c
4) b
5) a
6) b
7) b
8) a
9) c
10) c

## Chapter 5

1) b
2) d
3) c
4) a
5) c
6) d
7) a
8) d
9) b
10) c

## Chapter 6

1) b
2) d
3) a
4) b
5) d
6) b
7) d
8) a
9) c
10) b

*Orthodontics for Dental Hygienists and Dental Therapists*, First Edition. Tina Raked.
© 2018 John Wiley & Sons Ltd. Published 2018 by John Wiley & Sons Ltd.
Companion website: www.wiley.com/go/raked/orthodontics_dental_hygienists

## Chapter 7

1) d
2) d
3) a
4) d
5) c
6) c
7) b
8) d
9) a
10) b

## Chapter 8

1) b
2) c
3) d
4) a
5) d
6) d
7) d
8) a
9) d
10) b

## Chapter 9

1) b
2) d
3) c
4) a

5) a
6) d
7) a
8) a
9) b
10) d

## Chapter 10

1) d
2) c
3) d
4) a
5) b
6) d
7) c
8) a
9) a
10) d

## Chapter 11

1) a
2) c
3) b
4) b
5) c
6) d
7) b
8) d
9) d
10) b

# Index

*Orthodontics for Dental Hygienists and Dental Therapists*, First Edition. Tina Raked.
© 2018 John Wiley & Sons Ltd. Published 2018 by John Wiley & Sons Ltd.
Companion website: www.wiley.com/go/raked/orthodontics_dental_hygienists